Dermatologic Epidemiology and Public Health

Guest Editor

ROBERT P. DELLAVALLE, MD, PhD, MSPH

DERMATOLOGIC CLINICS

www.derm.theclinics.com

Consulting Editor
BRUCE H. THIERS, MD

April 2009 • Volume 27 • Number 2

SAUNDERS an imprint of ELSEVIER, Inc.

W.B. SAUNDERS COMPANY
A Division of Elsevier Inc.

1600 John F. Kennedy Boulevard • Suite 1800 • Philadelphia, PA 19103-2899

http://www.theclinics.com

DERMATOLOGIC CLINICS Volume 27, Number 2
April 2009 ISSN 0733-8635, ISBN-13: 978-1-4377-0469-3, ISBN 10: 1-4377-0469-7

Editor: Carla Holloway
Developmental Editor: Donald Mumford

Dermatologic Clinics (ISSN 0733-8635) is published quarterly by Elsevier Inc., 360 Park Avenue South, New York, NY 10010-1710. Months of publication are January, April, July, and October. Business and editorial offices: 1600 John F. Kennedy Blvd., Suite 1800, Philadelphia, PA 19103-2899. Customer service office: 11830 Westline Drive, St. Louis, MO 63146. Periodicals postage paid at New York, NY, and additional mailing offices. Subscription prices are USD 274.00 per year for US individuals, USD 423.00 per year for US institutions, USD 321.00 per year for Canadian individuals, USD 506.00 per year for Canadian institutions, USD 376.00 per year for international individuals, USD 506.00 per year for international institutions, USD 131.00 per year for US students/residents, and USD 189.00 per year for Canadian and international students/residents. International air speed delivery is included in all *Clinics* subscription prices. All prices are subject to change without notice. **POSTMASTER:** Send address changes to *Dermatologic Clinics*, Elsevier Journals Customer Service, 11830 Westline Drive, St. Louis, MO 63146. **Customer Service: 1-800-654-2452 (US and Canada). From outside of the US and Canada, call 1-314-453-7041. Fax: 1-314-453-5170. For print support, e-mail: JournalsCustomer Service-usa@elsevier.com. For online support, e-mail: JournalsOnlineSupport-usa@elsevier.com.**

Reprints. For copies of 100 or more, of articles in this publication, please contact the Commercial Reprints Department, Elsevier Inc., 360 Park Avenue South, New York, New York 10010-1710. Tel.: (212) 633-3813; Fax: (212) 462-1935; Email: reprints@elsevier.com.

The *Dermatologic Clinics* is covered in *MEDLINE/PubMed (Index Medicus)*, *Current Contents/Clinical Medicine*, *Excerpta Medica*, *Chemical Abstracts*, and *ISI/BIOMED*.

Printed and bound in the United Kingdom
Transferred to Digital Print 2011

Contributors

GUEST EDITOR

ROBERT P. DELLAVALLE, MD, PhD, MSPH
Department of Dermatology, University of
Colorado Denver School of Medicine, Aurora,
Colorado; Dermatology Service, Department of
Veterans Affairs Medical Center, Denver,
Colorado; and Colorado School of Public Health,
Aurora, Colorado

AUTHORS

ADAM ASARCH, BA
Tufts University School of Medicine, Boston,
Massachusetts

MARIANNE BERWICK, PhD, MPH
Professor of Internal Medicine, Division of
Epidemiology and Biostatistics, Department
of Internal Medicine, University of New Mexico,
Albuquerque, New Mexico; and Associate
Director, Population Science, University of New
Mexico Cancer Center, Albuquerque, New Mexico

KRISTINE L. BUSSE, MS
Department of Dermatology, Wright State
University Boonshoft School of Medicine, Dayton,
Ohio

LILIANE CHATENOUD, ScBiol
Centro Studi Gruppo Italiano Studi Epidemiologici
in Dermatologia (GISED), Ospedali Riuniti,
Bergamo, Italy; and Department of Epidemiology,
Mario Negri Institute for Pharmacological
Research, Milan, Italy

ANNIE CHIU, MD
Cedars-Sinai Medical Group, Beverly Hills,
California

LORI A. CRANE, PhD, MPH
Colorado School of Public Health, Aurora,
Colorado; and University of Colorado at Denver
and Health Sciences Center, Denver, Colorado

ROBERT P. DELLAVALLE, MD, PhD, MSPH
Department of Dermatology, University of
Colorado Denver School of Medicine, Aurora,
Colorado; Dermatology Service, Department
of Veterans Affairs Medical Center, Denver,
Colorado; and Colorado School of Public Health,
Aurora, Colorado

CORY A. DUNNICK, MD
Assistant Professor of Dermatology, Department
of Dermatology, University of Colorado Denver,
Aurora, Colorado

JEFFREY I. ELLIS, MD
Clinical Instructor, SUNY Downstate Medical
Center; and Department of Medicine, Division
of Dermatology, North Shore/Long Island Jewish
Hospital, Plainview, New York

ESTHER ERDEI, PhD
Research Assistant Professor, Division of
Epidemiology and Biostatistics, Department
of Internal Medicine, University of New Mexico,
Albuquerque, New Mexico

STEVEN R. FELDMAN, MD, PhD
Professor of Dermatology, Pathology and Public
Health Sciences, Center for Dermatology
Research, Department of Dermatology;
Department of Pathology; and Division of Public
Health Sciences, Wake Forest University School
of Medicine, Winston-Salem, North Carolina

SCOTT R. FREEMAN, MD
Dermatology Resident, Department of
Dermatology, University of Colorado at Denver
Health Sciences Center, Aurora, Colorado

JENNIFER HAY, PhD
Assistant Attending Psychologist, Department
of Psychiatry and Behavioral Sciences, Memorial
Sloan-Kettering Cancer Center, New York,
New York

HEATHER E. HOCH, MS
Department of Dermatology, University of
Colorado Denver School of Medicine, Aurora,
Colorado

WILLIAM HOWE, MD
Department of Dermatology, University of
Colorado Denver, School of Medicine, Aurora,
Colorado

ALIREZA KHATAMI, MD, MSPH
Assistant Professor of Dermatology, Center for
Research and Training in Skin Diseases and
Leprosy, Tehran University of Medical Sciences,
Tehran, Iran

ALEXA B. KIMBALL, MD, MPH
Vice Chair, Department of Dermatology,
Massachusetts General Hospital; Associate
Professor, Harvard Medical School, Boston,
Massachusetts; and Director, Clinical Unit for
Research Trials in Skin (CURTIS), Massachusetts
General and Brigham and Women's Hospitals,
Boston, Massachusetts

YAKIR S. LEVIN, PhD
Stanford University Schools of Medicine and
Engineering, Palo Alto, California

LINH K. LU, MD, PhD
Staff Physician, Southern California Permanente
Medical Group, Fontana, California

LUIGI NALDI, MD
Centro Studi Gruppo Italiano Studi Epidemiologici
in Dermatologia (GISED), Department of
Dermatology, Ospedali Riuniti, Bergamo, Italy

CHRISTINA A. NELSON, MD
Preventive Medicine Resident, Department of
Preventive Medicine and Biometrics, University of
Colorado at Denver Health Sciences Center
(UCHSC), Denver, Colorado

TAMAR NIJSTEN, MD, PhD
Department of Dermatology, Erasmus Medical
Center, Rotterdam, The Netherlands

BRIDGIT V. NOLAN, BA
Medical Student, SUNY Upstate Medical
University, Syracuse, New York

MIGUEL SAN SEBASTIAN, MD, PhD
Associate Professor, Department of Public Health
and Clinical Medicine, Epidemiology and Public
Health Sciences, Umeå International School of
Public Health, Umeå University, Umeå, Sweden

ANGELA SAUAIA, MD, PhD
Associate Professor, Division of Health Care Policy
and Research, Department of Medicine, University
of Colorado Denver School of Medicine; and
Associate Professor, Department of Surgery,
University of Colorado Denver School of Medicine,
Aurora, Colorado

RACHEL N. SIMMONS, BS
Medical Student, University of Florida College
of Medicine, Gainesville, Florida

RAJA K. SIVAMANI, MS
University of California, Davis, School of Medicine,
Sacramento, California

KARL VANCE, BS
Department of Dermatology, University of
Colorado Denver, School of Medicine, Aurora,
Colorado

MARLIES WAKKEE, MD
Department of Dermatology, Erasmus Medical
Center, Rotterdam, Netherlands

ERIN M. WARSHAW, MD, MS
Associate Professor of Dermatology, University
of Minnesota; and Chief of Dermatology,
Minneapolis Veterans Affairs Medical Center,
Minneapolis, Minnesota

Contents

Preface   xi

Robert P. Dellavalle

Dedication   xiii

Publisher's Note   xv

Skin Disease: A Neglected Public Health Problem   99

Alireza Khatami and Miguel San Sebastian

> Skin diseases are among the most common health problems in humans. Consider-
> ing their significant impact on the individual, the family, the social life of patients, and
> their heavy economical burden, the public health importance of these diseases is
> underappreciated. This article discusses the importance of dermatologic public
> health and makes recommendations for better addressing this neglected topic.

Health Care Inequities: An Introduction for Dermatology Providers   103

Angela Sauaia and Robert P. Dellavalle

> When differences in health and health care are avoidable and unfair, they are labeled
> health inequities. In large part health inequities reflect social determinants of health,
> lack of access to care, and a health care system that does not allow sufficient time
> and resources so high-quality care may be provided to all patients. Programs aiming
> at reducing health disparities must include the provision of services as well as ad-
> dress access to care and socioeconomic barriers. This article focuses on health
> care disparities in dermatology, and invites providers to become agents of change.

Ultraviolet Tanning Addiction   109

Bridgit V. Nolan and Steven R. Feldman

> Behavioral studies of ultraviolet light exposure behavior have provided insight into
> motivations for tanning, which include not only the desire for a tanned appearance
> but also the physiologic response to ultraviolet light. Many frequent tanners continue
> to tan despite knowledge or personal experience of adverse consequences. Efforts
> to reduce tanning behavior need to account for the interplay between physiologic
> effects of tanning and psychosocial drives behind tanning behavior.

Dermatologic Medication Adherence   113

Bridgit V. Nolan and Steven R. Feldman

> Human behavior is directly related to the development of various skin disease con-
> ditions and to the effectiveness of skin disease treatment regimens. Adherence re-
> search studies have demonstrated abysmal adherence to topical treatment of
> common skin disorders, opening new opportunities for improving skin disease treat-
> ment outcomes. The treatment of skin raises unique issues in environmental expo-
> sures, psychosocial human interactions, biology, and pharmacology. The resulting
> human behaviors and the potential to understand and modify those behaviors
> through behavioral research studies are exciting and promising.

Survey Research in Dermatology: Guidelines for Success   121

Adam Asarch, Annie Chiu, Alexa B. Kimball, and Robert P. Dellavalle

> Survey research has been used to investigate a wide range of issues in dermatology. The proper use of survey design and analysis is critical for achieving reliable, accurate data and high impact in the medical literature. Here we describe the use of surveys from both a theoretical and practical standpoint. We provide recommendations for limiting error and producing interpretable results, followed by an outline for achieving publication. We conclude with a discussion of previous successful uses of survey studies in dermatologic literature.

Social Internet Sites as a Source of Public Health Information   133

Karl Vance, William Howe, and Robert P. Dellavalle

> Social media websites, such as YouTube, Facebook, MySpace, Twitter, and Second Life® are rapidly emerging as popular sources of health information especially for teens and young adults. Social media marketing carries the advantages of low cost, rapid transmission through a wide community, and user interaction. Disadvantages include blind authorship, lack of source citation, and presentation of opinion as fact. Dermatologists and other health care providers should recognize the importance of social media websites and their potential usefulness for disseminating health information.

Comorbidities in Dermatology   137

Marlies Wakkee and Tamar Nijsten

> Recently, comorbidities have been rediscovered in dermatology. Although numerous associations between skin diseases and other conditions have been reported, only a few are well documented. The association of comorbidities and dermatoses is complex and multifactorial. Life-style factors, impaired health-related quality of life, depression, therapeutic interventions, and several biases may confound the relationship between skin diseases and comorbidities. This article discusses observational studies that assess comorbidities in psoriasis, atopic dermatitis, vitiligo, and nonmelanoma skin cancer, and the likelihood of the observed associations and their clinical consequences.

The Benefits and Risks of Ultraviolet Tanning and Its Alternatives: The Role of Prudent Sun Exposure   149

Raja K. Sivamani, Lori A. Crane, and Robert P. Dellavalle

> Sunlight- and indoor ultraviolet (UV)-induced tanning is a common behavior, especially among adolescents, young adults, and individuals who have lighter skin. Excessive sun exposure is associated with several health risks, including the acceleration of skin aging and the promotion of skin cancers. Several health benefits of UV exposure include vitamin D production and improved mood. This article analyzes these health risks and benefits and discusses pertinent issues surrounding indoor tanning, the role of sunless tanning products, and prudent sun exposure.

Prevention of Nickel Allergy: The Case for Regulation?   155

Linh K. Lu, Erin M. Warshaw, and Cory A. Dunnick

> Nickel is the most common allergen detected in patch-tested patients. Nickel allergy is highest among females and patients under the age of 18, affecting 35.8% of

patients patch-tested in this demographic. Nickel allergic contact dermatitis is a T-cell–mediated immune reaction which most commonly presents as a skin rash in areas exposed to nickel; however, more serious reactions to nickel in medical devices and more widespread eruptions to dietary nickel can occur. In contrast to Europe, where regulations have resulted in a decreasing prevalence of nickel allergy, the incidence of nickel allergic contact dermatitis in North America is increasing. This article summarizes primary prevention strategies as well as management of patients already sensitized to nickel.

Teledermatology: A Review of Reliability and Accuracy of Diagnosis and Management   163

Yakir S. Levin and Erin M. Warshaw

In this article, the authors summarize the published literature on the reliability and accuracy of teledermatology. The first section reports on the diagnostic reliability of teledermatology compared with face-to-face clinic consultation. In the second section, the authors report on the "intragroup" diagnostic agreement between either clinic dermatologists or teledermatologists. The third section discusses the diagnostic accuracy for those studies that include definitive histopathologic diagnosis. The last section summarizes the literature comparing clinical management decisions by clinic dermatologists to those made by teledermatologists.

Consumer Empowerment in Dermatology   177

Heather E. Hoch, Kristine L. Busse, and Robert P. Dellavalle

Health care consumers increasingly confront and collaborate with medical providers. This article describes recent developments in health care consumer activism including dermatology disease advocacy and efforts to improve dermatologist-patient interactions.

Registry Research in Dermatology   185

Luigi Naldi and Liliane Chatenoud

A medical "registry" is a systematic collection of information from cases of a particular disease or other health relevant condition. Hospital-based registries primarily address prognosis, whereas population-based registries provide estimates of disease incidence. Opportunities to establish and investigate dermatology hospital- and population-based registries abound.

Dermatology Internet Resources   193

Rachel N. Simmons, Jeffrey I. Ellis, and Robert P. Dellavalle

Many Internet resources for dermatologists benefit public health by providing education and information on the diagnosis and treatment of skin conditions. A variety of dermatology resources exist on the Web, but finding quality resources can be time-consuming. The authors provide a collection of high-quality, freely accessible, English-language Web sites that they have categorized as clinical, educational, or evidence-based medicine resources. They hope that this list of sources helps to meet the informational needs of dermatologists and promotes skin disease awareness and education.

Reviewing Dermatology Manuscripts and Publications 201

Christina A. Nelson, Scott R. Freeman, and Robert P. Dellavalle

Although quality scientific publications depend on peer review, physicians rarely receive formal training on how to review a manuscript. Comprehensive guidelines direct how meta-analyses, randomized controlled trials (RTCs), and observational trials should be reported in the literature. This article provides instruction on how to effectively review a life sciences manuscript, particularly those in dermatology.

Melanoma Epidemiology and Public Health 205

Marianne Berwick, Esther Erdei, and Jennifer Hay

This article reviews the research on, and examines the epidemiology and prevention of melanoma. Despite the great quantity of research into environmental and genetic causes, and the ease of diagnosis, incidence and mortality have risen in all developed countries during the last half century. Patient and physician education, and public health programs aimed at prevention, have had varied success. The authors conclude that, until we have better data on how to prevent skin cancer of all types, the best solutions are education of high-risk populations about skin self-evaluation in combination with physician examination to practice; and sun protection.

Index 215

Dermatologic Clinics

FORTHCOMING ISSUES

July 2009

Cosmetic Dermatology
Vic Narukar, MD, *Guest Editor*

October 2009

Contact Dermatitis
Susan Nedorost, MD, *Guest Editor*

January 2010

**Epidermolysis Bullosa: Pathogenesis, Diagnosis,
and Management—Part I**
Dedee Murrell, MD,
Guest Editor

RECENT ISSUES

January 2009

Antibiotic Use in Dermatology
James Q. Del Rosso, DO, FAOCD,
Guest Editor

October 2008

Panniculitis
Luis Requena, MD, *Guest Editor*

July 2008

Spa Dermatology
Neil S. Sadick, MD, *Guest Editor*

RELATED INTEREST

Dermatologic Clinics April 2008 (Volume 26, Issue 2)
International Dermatology
Torello Lotti, MD, *Guest Editor*
www.derm.theclinics.com

THE CLINICS ARE NOW AVAILABLE ONLINE!

Access your subscription at:
www.theclinics.com

Preface

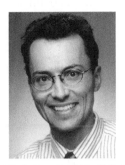

Robert P. Dellavalle, MD, PhD, MSPH
Guest Editor

This odyssey began with an email from Bruce Theirs asking me to consider editing a special issue of *Dermatologic Clinics* dedicated to dermatoepidemiology. We quickly decided to broaden the focus to include public health, making this the first issue of any *Clinics of North America* series specifically devoted to the topic of public health. I solicited potential articles from colleagues and members of the dermatoepidemiology list serve maintained by Martin Weinstock at Brown University (Providence, Rhode Island). Articles were submitted and peer reviews done in the fall of 2008. Reviewers were given the option of revealing or not revealing their identity to the authors and to our readers. I thank the peer reviewers listed below for their attention to detail, and for the hundreds of comments they offered that have vastly improved this issue: Adam Asarch (two articles), Maged Kamel Boulos, David Buller, Avanta Collier, Lori Crane (three articles), Guy Eslick, Rod Hay, Whitney High, Alexa Kimball, Kristie McNealy (two articles), David Norris, Rachael Simmons, Hywel Williams (two articles), and others who remain anonymous.

Although hot-button issues in both fields are discussed, the articles, in the end, treat dermatologic public health topics more than epidemiology. Alireza Khatami and Miguel San Sebastian lead off this issue discussing the community health perspective on skin disease as a neglected public health problem. Angela Sauaia and I next address disparities in dermatologic health care. Bridgit Nolan and Steven Feldman review behavioral study topics particularly relevant to dermatology: tanning addiction and medication compliance. Adam Asarch and colleagues summarize the principles of sound survey research. Karl Vance and colleagues describe the potential of social website marketing for dermatologic public health messages. Marlies Wakkee and Tamar Nijsten review the increasing importance of comorbidities in dermatologic research. Raja Sivamani and colleagues examine ultraviolet tanning public health messaging. Linh Lu and colleagues make the case for increased nickel regulation to reduce the most common cause of allergic contact dermatitis. Yakir Levin and Erin Warshaw review the emerging field of teledermatology. Heather Hoch and colleagues expose the growing influence of health care consumers on dermatology. Luigi Naldi and Liliane Chatenoud describe registry research examples, opportunities, and pitfalls, and provide guidelines for the reporting of this type of research. Rachel Simmons and colleagues describe online dermatology resources. Christina Neslon and colleagues suggest guidelines for manuscript and publication review. And, lastly, Marianne Berwick and colleagues outline the epidemiology and public health issues of one of dermatology's gravest problems—melanoma.

This issue of *Dermatologic Clinics* also initiates one of the first uses of podcasts[1] by a dermatology journal. I thank Chis Mavergames and Mike Clark for teaching an exciting workshop on the importance of this new technology at the Cochrane

Supported by University of Colorado Denver, School of Medicine Colorado Health Informatics Collaboration interdisciplinary academic enrichment funds (RPD) and by National Cancer Institute (NCI) grant K-07 CA92550.

Dermatol Clin 27 (2009) xi–xii
doi:10.1016/j.det.2008.12.003
0733-8635/08/$ – see front matter. Published by Elsevier Inc.

Colloquium in Freiberg, Germany, in October of 2008.

I thank Bruce Theirs for the invitation to edit this issue. I thank Carla Holloway for her professional editorial assistance. I thank the University of Colorado Denver, School of Medicine for interdisciplinary academic enrichment funds that supported discussion sessions among some of the authors, and the National Cancer Institute for a career development grant that supported some of my salary while working on this project. And lastly, I thank my wife, Lisa, and my children, Natalia and Eric, for accommodating the time and effort this project directed away from their company and love.

Robert P. Dellavalle, MD, PhD, MSPH
Colorado School of Public Health
13001 E. 17th Place
Campus Box B119
Aurora, CO, 80045, USA

E-mail address:
Robert.Dellavalle@ucdenver.edu (R.P. Dellavalle)

REFERENCE

1 Morris T, Tomasi C, Terra E, et al. Podcasting for Dummies. 2nd edition. New York: Wiley Publishing; 2008.

Dedication

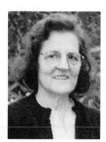

I dedicate this issue to my aunt and godmother Luciana Dellavalle who died during the production of this issue; I will always remember her delicious cooking, Tuscan proverbi, and deep religious faith.

Robert P. Dellavalle

Dermatol Clin 27 (2009) xiii
doi:10.1016/j.det.2009.02.001
0733-8635/09/$ – see front matter © 2009 Published by Elsevier Inc.

Publisher's Note

Podcasts for this issue of *Dermatologic Clinics* are available at www.derm.theclinics.com

Dermatol Clin 27 (2009) xv
doi:10.1016/j.det.2009.02.002
0733-8635/09/$ – see front matter

Skin Disease: A Neglected Public Health Problem

Alireza Khatami, MD, MSPH[a],*, Miguel San Sebastian, MD, PhD[b]

KEYWORDS

- Dermatology • Public health • Burden of illness
- Acne vulgaris • Dermatitis • Herpes simplex
- Herpes zoster • Primary health care

PUBLIC HEALTH PERSPECTIVE

The World Health Organization (WHO) produced a comprehensive global health plan more than 2 decades ago entitled "Health for All by the Year 2000." Tellingly, although this optimistic plan predicated a level of health necessary for socially and economically productive lives, it neglected dermatologic health.[1]

The *New Oxford Dictionary of English* defines dermatology as "the branch of medicine concerned with the diagnosis and treatment of skin diseases."[2] In practice, dermatology includes about 3000 diseases that affect the skin and its appendages (eg, hair and nails).[3] While many notorious epidemics with prominent skin manifestations of ages past, such as small pox, plague, leprosy, and anthrax, have been quelled,[4] other dermatologic diseases such as genital warts, acne, and dermatitis remain exceedingly common. For example, in 2004, more than half (165 million) of the US population suffered from herpes simplex virus (HSV) and herpes zoster virus (HZV) infections, and 83.3 million cases of human papilloma virus (HPV) infection occurred.[3] Indeed, at any given time, one fourth of us (or more) suffer from at least one skin disease[2,5,6]—a situation that constitutes a significant global burden of disease.[2,3,7–14]

BURDEN OF DISEASE

The total economical burden of skin diseases (inclusive for economical burden on the quality of life) was estimated at 96 billion US dollars in 2004.[3] The visibility of dermatologic illness increases this burden; disfigurement and social handicap are commonly reported by patients with skin disease.[15] Skin diseases can reduce family income (eg, reduction of wages caused by the inability to work) and increase expenditures (eg, extra payments for health service and prescriptions). Skin disease also causes mortality—the mortality rate for skin disease in Sub-Saharan Africa was comparable to that of hepatitis B, meningitis, obstructed delivery, and rheumatic heart disease. In addition, disability-adjusted life years (DALYs) equaled 896,000 for the same region which is comparable to gout, endocrine disorders, panic disorders, and war-related injuries.[11] Better information sources and proper instruments for correct measurement of prevalence of skin diseases, their impact on patient quality of life, and their economical burden are needed.[16]

DERMATOLOGIC PUBLIC HEALTH NEGLECT

The low-mortality rate of the majority of skin diseases, in comparison with other diseases,

This work was presented orally at the *21st World Congress of Dermatology* in Buenos Aires, Argentina, in the "Interactive Epidemiology" session on October 5, 2007.

[a] Center for Research and Training in Skin Diseases and Leprosy, No. 79, Taleqani Avenue, Tehran 14166-13675, Iran
[b] Department of Public Health and Clinical Medicine, Epidemiology and Public Health Sciences, Umeå International School of Public Health, Umeå University, SE-901 85 Umeå, Sweden
* Corresponding author.
E-mail address: akhatami@tums.ac.ir (A. Khatami).

Dermatol Clin 27 (2009) 99–101
doi:10.1016/j.det.2008.11.011

may cause international health policymakers and local decision makers to make them a low priority.[7,11,17,18] Primary care providers who have not been specially trained might be unable to diagnose skin conditions correctly.[11] Some populations with high prevalence of dermatologic conditions are not easily accessible, especially the poor, elderly, and immigrants.[6,19] Finally, the benefits of public health interventions in reducing the prevalence, morbidity, and mortality of skin diseases may be underestimated. An example of the importance of this work is the decrease in melanoma mortality and incidence rates among younger cohorts in Australia due to sun safety health education.[20]

PRIMARY HEALTH CARE: A NEW OPPORTUNITY

The World Health Report 2008 will focus on the role of primary health care in strengthening health systems. Global health networks, such as the Peoplés Health Movement, have been calling for a revitalization of the principles of the Alma-Ata Declaration where primary health care should guarantee universal access to quality health care.[21] New initiatives seek to invest 15% of the budget of vertical disease-oriented programs in strengthening well-coordinated, integrated, local primary health care systems.[22] Given the importance of integrating curative and preventive care of dermatologic diseases into local health facilities, the revitalization of primary health care could provide a means to raise dermatologic conditions higher in the international public health agenda.

To this end, we recommend that all parties interested in fostering dermatologic public health:

- Acknowledge that dermatologic illness creates significant quality of life, social, and economic burdens.
- Prioritize strategies for addressing dermatologic conditions at international and national levels.
- Conduct population-based surveys on representative samples to evaluate the prevalence of skin conditions and facilitate dermatologic needs assessment.
- Improve provider training in skin disease. (Even a one-day training program for health care providers in Mali improved their abilities in the diagnosis and treatment of common skin diseases and decreased the prescription costs.[23])
- Promote patient access and patient-physician referral systems to reduce undiagnosed and misdiagnosed skin diseases.
- Establish registries for specific skin diseases, particularly for those with a high-disease burden.
- Reduce hazardous occupational and leisure environmental exposures through education and interventions.

REFERENCES

1. Ryan TJ. Healthy skin for all. International Committee of Dermatology. Int J Dermatol 1994;33:829–35.
2. Burns DA, Cox NH. Introduction and historical bibliography. In: Breathnach S, Burns T, Griffiths C, editors. Rook's textbook of dermatology. 7th edition. Oxford: Blackwell Science; 2004. p. 1.
3. Bickers DR, Lim HW, Margolis D, et al. The burden of skin diseases: 2004 a joint project of the American Academy of Dermatology Association and the Society for Investigative Dermatology. J Am Acad Dermatol 2006;55:490–500.
4. Basch PF. Textbook of International Health. 2nd edition. New York: Oxford University Press; 1999.
5. Wolkenstein P, Grob JJ, Bastuji-Garin S, et al. Societe Francaise de Dermotologie. French people and skin diseases: results of a survey using a representative sample. Arch Dermatol 2003;139:1614–9.
6. Figueroa JI, Fuller LC, Abraha A, et al. Dermatology in the southwestern Ethiopia: rational for a community approach. Int J Dermatol 1998;37:752–8.
7. Chen SC, Bayoumi AM, Soon SL, et al. A catalog of dermatology utilities: a measure of the burden of skin diseases. J Investig Dermatol Symp Proc 2004;9:160–8.
8. Insinga RP, Dasbach EJ, Elbasha EH, et al. Assessing the annual economical burden of preventing and treating anogenital human papillomavirus-related disease in the US: analytic framework and review of the literature. Pharmacoeconomics 2005;23:1107–22.
9. Walker N, Lewis-Jones MS. Quality of life and acne in Scottish adolescent schoolchildren: use of the Children's Dermatology Life Quality Index (CDLQI) and the Cardiff Acne Disability Index (CADI). J Eur Acad Dermatol Venereol 2006;20:45–50.
10. Plunkett A, Merlin K, Gill D, et al. The frequency of common nonmalignant skin conditions in adults in central Victoria, Australia. Int J Dermatol 1999;38:901–8.
11. Hay R, Bendeck SE, Chen S, et al. Skin diseases. In: Jamison DT, Breman JG, Measham AR, editors. Disease control priorities in developing countries. 2nd edition. New York: Oxford University Press; 2006. p. 707–22.
12. Carroll CL, Balkrishnan R, Feldman SR, et al. The burden of atopic dermatitis: impact on the patient, family, and society. Pediatr Dermatol 2005;22:192–9.
13. Armstrong BK, Kricker A. The epidemiology of UV induced skin cancer. J Photochem Photobiol B 2001;63:8–18.

14. Ng JC, Wang J, Shraim A, et al. A global health problem caused by arsenic from natural sources. Chemosphere 2003;52:1353–9.

15. Johnson ML. Defining the burden of skin disease in the United States–a historical perspective. J Investig Dermatol Symp Proc 2004;9:108–10.

16. VanBeek M, Beach S, Braslow L, et al. Highlights from the report of the working group on "Core measures of the burden of skin diseases". J Invest Dermatol 2007;127:2701–6.

17. World Health Report 1998. Available at: http://www.who.int/whr/1998/en/whr98_en.pdf. Accessed November 7, 2006.

18. World Health Report 2006. Available at: http://www.who.int/whr/2006/whr06_en.pdf. Accessed November 9, 2006.

19. Marks R. Campaigning for melanoma prevention: a model for a health education program. J Eur Acad Dermatol Venereol 2004;18:44–7.

20. Morrone A, Toma L, Franco G, et al. Skin diseases highlighting essential global public health priorities. Int J Dermatol 2005;44:384–90.

21. Peoplés Health Movement. Available at: http://www.phmovement.org. Accessed February 1, 2007.

22. De Maeseneer J, van Weel C, Egilman D, et al. Strengthening primary care: addressing the disparity between vertical and horizontal investment. Br J Gen Pract 2008;8:3–4.

23. Mahé A, Faye O, N'Diaye HT, et al. Integration of basic dermatological care into primary health care services in Mali. Bull World Health Organ 2005;83:935–41.

Health Care Inequities: An Introduction for Dermatology Providers

Angela Sauaia, MD, PhD[a,b,]*, Robert P. Dellavalle, MD, PhD, MSPH[c,d,e]

KEYWORDS

- Health disparities • Minorities • Poverty • Melanoma
- Social determinants of health

Does our clinical practice acknowledge what we already know—namely, that social and environmental forces will limit the effectiveness of our treatments? Asking these questions needs to be the beginning of a conversation within medicine and public health, rather than the end of one.
— Paul Farmer, MD, PhD[1]

Racial and ethnic minorities, now about one third of the United States population, are expected to become the majority in 2042. By 2023, minorities will comprise more than half of all children,[2] and if the status quo is maintained, these children will live shorter, more painful and difficult lives than other children.[3,4]

The World Health Organization defines inequities as unfair systematic differences in health judged avoidable by reasonable action.[5] This article focuses not on the presentation of cutaneous diseases among people with different skin colors[6–13] but instead on health care disparities in dermatology, and invites providers to become agents of change.

HEALTH DISPARITIES IN THE UNITED STATES

The United States has long recognized the existence of health disparities. Since 2003, the Agency for Healthcare Research and Quality has produced the annual National Health Disparities Report in response to a legislative mandate from the US Congress.[3] The 2007 National Health Disparities Report noted that many of the largest gaps in health care quality and access have not diminished and emphasized the persistent lack of health insurance as a major barrier to reducing disparities.[3]

Over 45 million individuals lack health insurance coverage in the United States, according to 2007 data of the Current Population Survey.[14] Minorities are more likely to be uninsured (Current Population Survey 2007 data: Latinos, 32.1%; blacks, 19.5%; Asians and Pacific Islanders, 16.8%) than whites (10.4%), and these percentages have remained steady for over 10 years (**Fig. 1**). Children are also affected: the Urban Institute and Kaiser Commission on Medicaid and the Uninsured analysis of the 2007 Current Population Survey shows that 8% of the white non-Latino children are

The authors report no financial conflicts. Dr. Sauaia received no support for writing this article. Dr. Dellavalle's work was supported by the University of Colorado Denver School of Medicine Colorado Health Informatics Collaboration interdisciplinary academic enrichment funds (RPD) and by a National Cancer Institute grant K-07 CA92550 (RPD).

a Division of Health Care Policy and Research, Department of Medicine, University of Colorado Denver School of Medicine, 13611 East Colfax Avenue, Suite 100, Aurora, CO 80045, USA
b Division of Cardiothoracic Surgery, Department of Surgery, University of Colorado Denver School of Medicine, 12631 E. 17th Avenue, L15-6602, MS C310 P.O. Box 6511, Aurora, CO 80045, USA
c Dermatology Service, Department of Veterans Affairs Medical Center, 1055 Clermont Street, #165, Denver, CO 80220, USA
d Department of Dermatology, University of Colorado Denver School of Medicine, P.O. Box 6511, Mail Stop 8127, Aurora, CO 80045, USA
e Colorado School of Public Health, 13001 E. 17th Place, Campus Box B119, Aurora, CO 80045, USA
* Corresponding author. Division of Health Care Policy and Research, Department of Medicine, University of Colorado Denver School of Medicine, 13611 East Colfax Avenue, Suite 100, Aurora, CO 80045.
E-mail address: angela.sauaia@ucdenver.edu (A. Sauaia).

Dermatol Clin 27 (2009) 103–107
doi:10.1016/j.det.2008.12.001

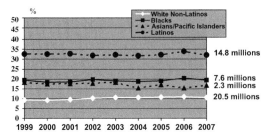

Fig. 1. National health insurance uninsured rates by racial and ethnic groups, 1999–2007. (*Data from* US Census Bureau, Current Population Survey, Annual Social and Economic Supplements [denominator: civilian non-institutional population].)

uninsured compared with 23% and 15% of the children in Latino and black populations.[15]

United States health insurance rates reflect income levels, and racial and ethnic minorities are more likely to be poor (12% of white non-Latinos are below the 100% Federal Poverty Level, compared with 29% of Latinos and 33% of blacks).[15] Social determinants of health include income and other closely related factors, such as housing, employment, environmental hazards, nutrition, discrimination, racism, and sexism.[1,5] These factors explain much of the observed differences in health care access and quality and predispose to poor health in the first place. Dermatology, like all fields of medicine, exhibits disparities.[7,16,17]

INEQUITIES IN SKIN CANCERS

The association of melanoma with lighter skin is reflected in the wide difference in age-adjusted incidence rates between racial groups. Data from the National Cancer Institute Surveillance Epidemiology and End Results 2001 to 2005 show that the invasive melanoma rate per 100,000 persons is 26.6 for whites, much higher than the observed numbers among blacks (1.0); Asians and Pacific Islanders (1.4); Native Americans and Alaska Natives (3.1); and Latinos (4.7).[18] The differences in age-adjusted mortality rates per 100,000 persons were less accentuated, with white non-Latinos rates of 3.3 compared with 0.4 in blacks and Asians and Pacific Islanders, 0.8 in Native Americans and Alaska Natives, and 0.7 in Latinos. Blacks with melanoma have lower survival rates compared with whites.[7]

The difference in mortality could be caused by differences in disease stage at time of diagnosis, which directly relates to access to care. Surveillance Epidemiology and End Results data from 1992 to 2002 revealed that melanoma was diagnosed at a later stage in minorities (blacks, 52.2%; Asian and Pacific Islanders, 57.4%; Latinos, 60.2%; Native Americans, 69.2%)

compared with whites (79.3%).[18,19] A Florida study reported a similar trend in tumor stage disparities among Latinos (localized disease Latinos, 74%, versus whites, 84%).[20] Data from the California Cancer Registry (1993–2003) revealed that low socioeconomic status was an independent predictor of survival after adjustments for age, sex, histology, stage, anatomic site, treatment, and race and ethnicity.[21] Although the crude disparity was reduced for all minority groups after adjustment for the other risk factors, a statistically significant increased risk of death remained for blacks compared with white non-Latinos (hazard ratio, 1.60; 95% confidence interval, 1.17–2.18), suggesting socioeconomic status explained some of the disparity.

Other factors play a role in melanoma survival rates. Individuals with darkly pigmented skin tend to develop melanomas in non–sun-exposed sites (palmar, plantar, and mucosal surfaces).[7,22] They are also less likely than lightly pigmented individuals to be aware of skin cancer risks, use sun protection, and undergo full body skin examination.[7,23–25] Other skin cancers for which some evidence suggests that the worse prognosis observed among non-whites could be partially caused by advanced stage at presentation (rather than a more aggressive form of the disease) are cutaneous T-cell lymphoma and Kaposi's sarcoma.[7] Collectively, these findings suggest that efforts to diminish differences in survival rates should be directed at diagnosing skin cancers among minorities at earlier stages. This could be accomplished by improving access to care and increasing awareness with culturally appropriate health education.

Any additional burden especially in the primary care setting poses a daunting challenge.[26] The disadvantaged, among whom minorities are disproportionately represented, because of poorer health, literacy, and language barriers, require extra time and effort from providers.[26] Health care reforms need to address the social determinants of health that directly influence prevention, screening, early diagnosis, and treatment.[5,21,27–29]

SOLUTIONS FOR HEALTH INEQUITIES

In addition to culturally competent education and health promotion, programs for reducing disparities must expand health services for the underserved.[30] Improved access to care includes health insurance, transportation, child care, time off from work, affordable copayments, and decreased language and literacy barriers. For example, offering evening and weekend clinic hours improves access to care for employed individuals, allowing them to attend appointments without missing work.

Interventions with patient navigators, accompagnateurs, and promoteras(es) show effectiveness, including testing in randomized clinical trials.[1,31-35] These workers are trained to assist community members in accessing and navigating the health care system. They can counsel patients about a number of prevention related issues (eg, sun protection), allowing physicians to focus on health issues that demand more technical expertise.[26] Despite its effectiveness, medical students, health care providers, and policy makers may be unaware of this resource.

The use of professional (as opposed to ad hoc) interpreters is associated with raising the quality of clinical care for limited English proficiency patients to levels comparable with patients without language barriers.[36] Although legal mandates provide for interpreters, financial constraints, lack of unawareness regarding the advantages of this resource, and the dangers of using family members (especially children) have hampered implementation.[37,38] Language line services provide an alternative approach for overcoming language barriers. For more information on the national standards (National Standards on Culturally and Linguistically Appropriate Services), see the Web site of the Office of Minority Health at http://www.omhrc.gov/.

As different cultures continue to enrich the country, dermatologists are more likely to face differences in communication, decision styles, values, and belief systems.[39] Cross-cultural communication models are also useful tools in assisting providers to understand better the patient's perspective.[40-46] These models stress the value of the uniqueness of each patient and patient-physician relationship. Patients who identify with a specific ethnic group do not all behave the same and do not all have the same beliefs. For a guiding principle from patient to patient, and from moment to moment for each patient, never assume their perspective; instead, ask them to describe it.

Educational resources need to follow the pace of changing demographics. Ethnic skin issue coverage at national meetings and in photographs in the major dermatology resources is limited.[47] More extensive information describing common and serious skin diseases in people of color in educational resources has been recommended.[47]

Provider cultural competency training highlighting health equity is another component of the solution.[48] Ideally, this training should be integrated into the professional curricula as opposed to delivered only in separate sessions.[48] Recently, the Society of General Internal Medicine Health Disparities Task Force published curriculum recommendations to (1) examine and understand attitudes, such as mistrust, subconscious bias, and stereotyping, which practitioners and patients may bring to clinical encounters; (2) gain knowledge of the existence and magnitude of health disparities, including the multifactorial causes of health disparities and the many solutions required to diminish or eliminate them; and (3) acquire the skills to communicate and negotiate effectively across cultures, languages, and literacy levels, including the use of key tools to improve communication.[49] The broad goal of a curriculum on health disparities is to foster provider commitment to addressing inequities.

The National Institute of Arthritis and Musculoskeletal and Skin Diseases included reducing disparities as part of its Long Range Plan for 2006 to 2009.[16] This plan includes supporting research at institutions with substantial minority enrollment and participation in National Institutes of Health programs for underrepresented minority investigators and collaboration with minority-serving organizations (National Medical Association, the Association of Minority Health Professions Schools, and the Student National Medical Association) to increase the recruitment of underrepresented minority to research careers. The American Academy of Dermatology invites medical students from ethnically and socioeconomically diverse groups to participate in the Academy's Diversity Mentorship Program (http://www.aad.org/education/students/students.html).

Recently, a study using data from the National Ambulatory Medical Care Survey reported "in the United States, Blacks and Asians/Pacific Islanders are more likely than Whites to seek medical care for atopic dermatitis."[50] The information was not conducive to a suitable intervention because any intervention directed to such a heterogeneous group of peoples was unlikely to help.[51] Another issue is the relationship between race and skin color.[52] The relationship between skin color and ancestry has been shown to be quite variable, underscoring the need for caution when using pigmentation as a proxy of ancestry or when extrapolating the results from one admixed population to another.[53-57]

The variable race is not a biological construct that reflects innate differences, but a social construct that precisely captures the impacts of racism.

—Camara P. Jones, MD[58]

Recommendations of a 1994 National Institutes of Health–sponsored conference on measuring social inequalities in health in the United States included among others (1) routinely present data by socioeconomic position in conjunction with data on gender, race, ethnicity, and age; (2) conduct research to ensure that socioeconomic measures are valid for analyzing inequalities in health among women, children, older people, and diverse ethnic groups; and (3) use a core set of socioeconomic measures in all data bases to permit comparison of results across time.[59]

SUMMARY

When differences in health and health care are avoidable and unfair, they are labeled health inequities. In large part health inequities reflect social determinants of health, lack of access to care, and a health care system that does not allow sufficient time and resources so that high-quality care may be provided to all patients. Melanoma, cutaneous T-cell lymphoma, and possibly Kaposi's sarcoma are among the cutaneous diseases that have been associated with worse prognosis in minorities in large part because of presentation at advanced stages. Programs aiming at reducing health disparities must include the provision of services as well as address access to care and socioeconomic barriers.

REFERENCES

1. Farmer PE, Nizeye B, Stulac S, et al. Structural violence and clinical medicine. PLoS Med 2006; 3(10):e449.
2. US Census Bureau. US Census Bureau. 2008. Available at: www.census.gov. Accessed September 22, 2008.
3. 2007 National Health Care Disparities Report. Agency for Healthcare Research and Quality and Department of Health and Human Services. 2008. Available at: http://www.ahrq.gov/qual/qrdr07.htm. 2008; Accessed September 22, 2008.
4. Health, United States, 2007. Centers for Disease Control and Prevention, National Centers for Health Statistics. 2008. Available at: http://www.cdc.gov/nchs/hus.htm. Accessed September 22, 2008.
5. Closing the gap in one generation: health equity through action on the social determinants of health. World Health Organization Commission on Social Determinants of Health. 2008. Available at: http://www.who.int/social_determinants/final_report/en/index.html. Accessed September 22, 2008.
6. Cornelison RL Jr. Cutaneous diseases in Native Americans. Dermatol Clin 2003;21(4):699–702.
7. Gloster J, Neal K. Skin cancer in skin of color. J Am Acad Dermatol 2006;55(5):741–60.
8. Richards GM, Oresajo CO, Halder RM. Structure and function of ethnic skin and hair. Dermatol Clin 2003;21(4):595–600.
9. Halder RM, Nootheti PK. Ethnic skin disorders overview. J Am Acad Dermatol 2003;48(6 Suppl 1):S143–8.
10. Halder RM, Nandedkar MA, Neal KW. Pigmentary disorders in ethnic skin. Dermatol Clin 2003;21(4): 617–28, vii.
11. Sanchez MR. Cutaneous diseases in Latinos. Dermatol Clin 2003;21(4):689–97.
12. Halder RM, Roberts CI, Nootheti PK. Cutaneous diseases in the black races. Dermatol Clin 2003; 21(4):679–87, ix.
13. Lee CS, Lim HW. Cutaneous diseases in Asians. Dermatol Clin 2003;21(4):669–77.
14. Current Population Survey. Annual Social and Economic Supplements. US Census Bureau. 2008. Available at: http://www.census.gov/hhes/www/hlthins/. Accessed September 22, 2008.
15. Urban Institute and Kaiser Commission on Medicaid and the Uninsured analysis of the March 2007 Current Population Survey. Kaiser Family Foundation. 2008. Available at: http://www.kff.org/content/chartsdata.cfm. Accessed September 22, 2008.
16. Katz SI. Strategic plan for reducing health disparities. National Institute of Arthritis and Musculoskeletal and Skin Diseases. 2006. Available at: http://www.niams.nih.gov/About_Us/Mission_and_Purpose/strat_plan_hd.asp. Accessed August 15, 2008.
17. Bellows CF, Belafsky P, Fortgang IS, et al. Melanoma in African-Americans: trends in biological behavior and clinical characteristics over two decades. J Surg Oncol 2001;78(1):10–6.
18. Surveillance, epidemiology and end results. National Cancer Institute. 2008. Available at: http://seer.cancer.gov/. Accessed September 22, 2008.
19. Cormier JN, Xing Y, Ding M, et al. Ethnic differences among patients with cutaneous melanoma. Arch Intern Med 2006;166(17):1907–14.
20. Hu S, Soza-Vento RM, Parker DF, et al. Comparison of stage at diagnosis of melanoma among Hispanic, black, and white patients in Miami-Dade County, Florida. Arch Dermatol 2006;142(6):704–8.
21. Zell JA, Cinar P, Mobasher M, et al. Survival for patients with invasive cutaneous melanoma among ethnic groups: the effects of socioeconomic status and treatment. J Clin Oncol 2008;26(1):66–75.
22. Hu S, Ma F, Collado-Mesa F, et al. UV radiation, latitude, and melanoma in US Hispanics and blacks. Arch Dermatol 2004;140(7):819–24.
23. Ma F, Collado-Mesa F, Hu S, et al. Skin cancer awareness and sun protection behaviors in white Hispanic and white non-Hispanic high school students in Miami, Florida. Arch Dermatol 2007;143(8):983–8.
24. Pipitone M, Robinson JK, Camara C, et al. Skin cancer awareness in suburban employees: a Hispanic perspective. J Am Acad Dermatol 2002; 47(1):118–23.
25. Rodriguez GL, Ma F, Federman DG, et al. Predictors of skin cancer screening practice and attitudes in

primary care. J Am Acad Dermatol 2007;57(5): 775–81.

26. Fiscella K, Epstein RM. So much to do, so little time: care for the socially disadvantaged and the 15-minute visit. Arch Intern Med 2008;168(17):1843–52.

27. Peacey V, Steptoe A, Sanderman R, et al. Ten-year changes in sun protection behaviors and beliefs of young adults in 13 European countries. Prev Med 2006;43(6):460–5.

28. Reyes-Ortiz CA, Goodwin JS, Freeman JL, et al. Socio-economic status and survival in older patients with melanoma. J Am Geriatr Soc 2006;54(11):1758–64.

29. Mark PP. Predictors of sun protection in Canadian adults. Can J Public Health 2002;93(6):471–4.

30. Farmer PE. Pathologies of power: health, human rights, and the new war on the poor. 1st edition. Berkeley (CA): University of California Press; 2005.

31. Welsh AL, Sauaia A, Jacobellis J, et al. The effect of two church-based interventions on breast cancer screening rates among Medicaid-insured Latinas. Prev Chronic Dis 2005;2(4):A07 [Epub 2005 Sep 15].

32. Sauaia A, Min SJ, Lack D, et al. Church-based breast cancer screening education: impact of two approaches on Latinas enrolled in public and private health insurance plans. Prev Chronic Dis 2007;4(4):A99 [Epub 2007 Sep 15].

33. Fischer SM, Sauaia A, Kutner JS. Patient navigation: a culturally competent strategy to address disparities in palliative care. J Palliat Med 2007;10(5):1023–8.

34. Freeman HP. Patient navigation: a community based strategy to reduce cancer disparities. J Urban Health 2006;83(2):139–41.

35. Lina J, Yahaira G, Jaime L, et al. Use of a patient navigator to increase colorectal cancer screening in an urban neighborhood health clinic. J Urban Health 2005;82(2):216–24.

36. Karliner LS, Jacobs EA, Chen AH, et al. Do professional interpreters improve clinical care for patients with limited English proficiency? A systematic review of the literature. Health Serv Res 2007;42(2):727–54.

37. Lee KC, Winickoff JP, Kim MK, et al. Resident physicians' use of professional and nonprofessional interpreters: a national survey. JAMA 2006;296(9):1050–3.

38. Jacobs EA, Shepard DS, Suaya JA, et al. Overcoming language barriers in health care: costs and benefits of interpreter services. Am J Public Health 2004;94(5):866–9.

39. Moy JA, McKinley-Grant L, Sanchez MR. Cultural aspects in the treatment of patients with skin disease. Dermatol Clin 2003;21(4):733–42.

40. Kleinman A, Benson P. Anthropology in the clinic: the problem of cultural competency and how to fix it. PLoS Med 2006;3(10):e294.

41. Dobbie AE, Medrano M, Tysinger J, et al. The BELIEF instrument: a preclinical teaching tool to elicit patients' health beliefs. Fam Med 2003;35(5):316–9.

42. Berlin EA, Fowkes WC Jr. A teaching framework for cross-cultural health care: application in family practice. West J Med 1983;139(6):934–8.

43. Stuart MR, Leibermann JR. The fifteen minute hour: applied psychotherapy for the primary care physician. New York: Praeger; 1993.

44. Carrillo JE, Green AR, Betancourt JR. Cross-cultural primary care: a patient-based approach. Ann Intern Med 1999;130(10):829–34.

45. Betancourt JR, Carrillo JE, Green AR. Hypertension in multicultural and minority populations: linking communication to compliance. Curr Hypertens Rep 1999;1(6):482–8.

46. Green AR, Betancourt JR, Carrillo JE. Integrating social factors into cross-cultural medical education. Acad Med 2002;77(3):193–7.

47. Ebede T, Papier A. Disparities in dermatology educational resources. J Am Acad Dermatol 2006;55(4): 687–90.

48. Sauaia A, Fischer SM. Cultural competence training in medical schools: the quest for health equity. National Hispanic Medical Association 2006 Annual Meeting. 2006. Available at: http://www.nhmamd.org/presentationsummaries2007.htm. Accessed September 22, 2008.

49. Smith WR, Betancourt JR, Wynia MK, et al. Recommendations for teaching about racial and ethnic disparities in health and health care. Ann Intern Med 2007;147(9):654–65.

50. Janumpally SR, Feldman SR, Gupta AK, et al. In the United States, blacks and Asian/Pacific Islanders are more likely than whites to seek medical care for atopic dermatitis. Arch Dermatol 2002;138(5):634–7.

51. Williams HC. Have you ever seen an Asian/Pacific Islander? Arch Dermatol 2002;138(5):673–4.

52. Silver SE. Skin color is not the same thing as race. Arch Dermatol 2004;140(3):361.

53. Parra EJ, Kittles RA, Shriver MD. Implications of correlations between skin color and genetic ancestry for biomedical research. Nat Genet 2004; 36(Suppl 11):S54–60.

54. Bamshad M. Genetic influences on health: does race matter? JAMA 2005;294(8):937–46.

55. Cooper RS, Kaufman JS, Ward R. Race and genomics. N Engl J Med 2003;348(12):1166–70.

56. Tang H, Quertermous T, Rodriguez B, et al. Genetic structure, self-identified race/ethnicity, and confounding in case-control association studies. Am J Hum Genet 2005;76(2):268–75.

57. Williams HC. Race and ethnicity in dermatology. Arch Dermatol 2003;139:540.

58. Jones CP. Levels of racism: a theoretic framework and a gardener's tale. Am J Public Health 2000;90(8):1212–5.

59. Recommendations of the conference Measuring Social Inequalities in Health. Sponsored by the National Institutes of Health, September 28-30, 1994. Int J Health Serv 1996;26(3):521–7.

Ultraviolet Tanning Addiction

Bridgit V. Nolan, BA[a], Steven R. Feldman, MD, PhD[b],*

KEYWORDS

• Tanning • Ultraviolet • Addiction • Health services research

Human behavior has an intimate relationship to the development of skin disease. Skin is the protective organ at the interface with the environment and is the visual surface that humans present to the outside world. An intact epidermis, specifically the stratum corneum, is required for the skin to function as a physical and chemical barrier. Particular human behaviors, such as tanning and smoking, expose the skin to environmental risks and stress, which result in photoaging and skin cancer. Behavioral research is an exciting and growing area of dermatology. Research into risk-taking behavior, such as tanning, is flourishing, although perhaps not as quickly as in the areas of infectious diseases or substance abuse.

Skin cancer is the most common form of human cancer and its incidence is rising rapidly.[1] Exposure to ultraviolet radiation is the major avoidable risk factor for the development of melanoma and nonmelanoma skin cancer.[2] Despite evidence of the link between exposure to ultraviolet radiation and the development of skin cancer, exposure to ultraviolet radiation indoors and outdoors continues to increase.[3,4] The fact that frequent tanners are well informed about the risks for skin cancer and may be more knowledgeable than nontanning peers does not seem to influence their attitude or behavior.[5,6] This suggests that other factors operate in the continuance of tanning behavior.

Tanning is a high-risk behavior that may have addictive qualities. It has recently been noted that many tanners use ultraviolet light in excess of what is necessary for the desired tanned appearance. Tanning behavior exhibits signs of psychologic and physiologic dependence, and parallels exist between tanning behavior and other addictive syndromes.[6] Additional studies are needed to investigate more fully the issues of dependency and addiction associated with tanning.

INDOOR TANNING

Indoor tanning among young adults has increased from 1% to 27% between 1988 and 2007.[7] This trend has occurred in parallel with the increase in the perception that people look better with a tan and paradoxically with the increased awareness of the association between tanning and skin cancer.[7] Studies of tanning behavior among college students indicate that between 14% and 42% of these individuals engage in indoor tanning with prevalence rates higher among women.[6] The consistently identified top reasons for indoor tanning include an aesthetic preference for a tanned appearance, to "look better," and to experience associated relaxation and mood enhancement.[6] Recent survey studies investigating college students found that an overwhelming majority of past and current tanners (93% and 91%, respectively) believed that skin cancer is a possible consequence of using tanning beds.[5] Past and current tanners (81% and 52%, respectively) did not believe that tanning beds are safe.[5] Tanners know the dangers of tanning, but this does not deter them from engaging in high-risk behavior. Additionally, indoor tanning is associated with other behavioral health risk factors, such as smoking, recreational drug use, and eating disorders.[8]

In a large study (n = 29,294) investigating the prevalence and correlates of indoor tanning

The Center for Dermatology Research is supported by an unrestricted educational grant from Galderma Laboratories, L.P.

[a] SUNY Upstate Medical University, Weiskotten Hall, 766 Irving Avenue, Syracuse, NY 13210, USA
[b] Center for Dermatology Research, Wake Forest University School of Medicine, Medical Center Boulevard, Winston-Salem, NC 27157-1071, USA
* Corresponding author.
E-mail address: sfeldman@wfubmc.edu (S.R. Feldman).

Dermatol Clin 27 (2009) 109–112
doi:10.1016/j.det.2008.11.007

derm.theclinics.com

among the general adult population in the United States, the prevalence of indoor tanning was more common in individuals who were young, white, and female.[9] The overall prevalence of tanning was highest in individuals aged 18 to 29 (20.4%) and lowest among individuals over age 65 (7.8%).[9] A large study of French adults (n = 7200) attempted to characterize beliefs and behavior related to natural and artificial ultraviolet behavior. The most common reported justifications for tanning were aesthetic (30%) and in advance of vacation (37%).[10] The prevalence of indoor tanning within the study population was approximately 15%.[10] Tanning was significantly more prevalent among women than men (21% and 6%, respectively) with the frequency of indoor tanning greatest in the youngest age bracket.[10] Those who had fair skin and a history of sunburn events were more likely to use indoor tanning, supporting the association between fair phototype and desire for prevacation tan.[10] Smoking, another behavioral risk factor for the development of cancer, is more common among indoor tanners and these individuals are unconcerned about the risk for premature aging and skin cancer.[10]

EXISTING MODELS OF ADDICTION AND DEPENDENCE

Studies of frequent tanners have suggested possible links between tanning behavior and all established models of dependence and addiction. Social learning and cognitive models, pharmacologic models, behavioral models, and *Diagnostic and Statistical Manual*, Fourth Edition, Text Revision (*DSM*-IV-TR)-related models all have been used to study addiction and dependence.

According to the *DSM*-IV-TR, substance dependency is defined as having three or more of the following symptoms in a 12-month period: tolerance, withdrawal, difficulty controlling use, negative consequences, significant time or emotional energy spent, putting off or neglecting other activities, and desire to cut down.[11] Difficulty controlling use is relevant in that many tanners tan in excess of what is needed for the desired effect. Negative consequences in the form of acute sunburn, skin cancer, and premature aging also are present but knowledge of these factors does not deter frequent tanners. The pharmacologic model reinforces the concepts of physical and psychologic dependence, withdrawal, and tolerance as defining substance dependence. With repeated use of an agent, alterations in homeostatic set point occur, leading to physical dependence, which is characterized by tolerance and withdrawal.[12] A small, randomized controlled trial of

opioid antagonism in frequent and infrequent tanners tested whether or not opioid blockade produces withdrawal symptoms in frequent tanners. Results demonstrated that four of eight frequent tanners exhibited withdrawal symptoms consisting of nausea and jitteriness when given an opioid antagonist before ultraviolet exposure.[13] This effect was not observed in any of the infrequent tanners.[13] Psychologic dependence refers to the affect of a drug on the brain's reward system and its memory of the rewards. The production of sensations of pleasure or well-being encourages repeated use.[12] Many tanners report relaxation and mood-enhancing effects as motivation for tanning, suggesting the possibility of psychologic dependence.

Behavioral models of substance abuse emphasize positive reinforcing properties, substance recognition, and the association of environmental stimuli with substance use, and they differentiate addiction from other behaviors based on pathologic involvement, lack of control over the behavior, and continued use despite adverse effects.[14,15] Tanning has reinforcing properties and frequent tanners are able to distinguish between ultraviolet and nonultraviolet light-emitting tanning beds. Studies of high-risk tanning behavior among college undergraduates demonstrated continued use despite adverse personal experience, such as a blistering sunburn, and positive family history for skin cancer, and this association was stronger among individuals who scored positive on tanning-modified CAGE questionnaire.[6] CAGE questionnaire consist of four clinical questions used as a screening tool for detecting alcoholism: Have you ever felt you needed to Cut down on your drinking? Have people Annoyed you by criticizing your drinking? Have you ever felt Guilty about drinking? Have you ever felt you needed a drink first thing in the morning (Eye-opener) to steady your nerves or to get rid of a hangover?[16]

Important concepts related to social and cognitive learning models are outcome expectancy and self-efficacy.[17] Cluster analysis has shown that regular, year-round tanners have significantly more positive attitudes related to tanning.[18] Abstinence self-efficacy is a term used to describe an individual's belief in his or her ability to stop an activity.[17] Patients who have substance dependency show an inverse relationship between abstinence self-efficacy and level of dependence. In adolescents who tan, age of initiation and frequency of use correlated with difficulty quitting.[1] Individuals who were 13 years or younger at age of initiation were more likely to report difficulty quitting indoor tanning than individuals who were 16 to 17 years old at age of initiation (odds ratio 4.3; 95% CI, 1.3–14.7), and there was a statistically significant positive correlation between frequency of use and difficulty quitting indoor tanning.[1] Early age of initiation and frequency are correlated with alcohol and nicotine dependency, supporting the hypothesis that indoor tanning behavior may constitute a form of dependency.

SURVEY STUDIES SUGGESTING ULTRAVIOLET TANNING DEPENDENCE AND ADDICTION

Tanning behavior may be generated by an ultraviolet light substance-related disorder (SRD) in which repeated use leads to a behavior pattern similar to other types of substance dependence. A survey study of beachgoers (n = 145) using SRD criteria from the *DSM*-IV-TR and a tanning-modified CAGE questionnaire evaluated whether or not ultraviolet light constitutes a type of SRD.[19] Analysis demonstrated that 26% met tanning-modified CAGE criteria and that 53% met tanning-modified *DSM*-IV-TR diagnosis for SRD with respect to ultraviolet light tanning.[19] Results from another study using tanning-modified CAGE criteria to assess the prevalence of ultraviolet light SRD demonstrated that 12% of college undergraduates (n = 358) met tanning-modified CAGE criteria.[6] Women, individuals identified as indoor tanners, frequent tanners, and students who had family and friends who also tan were more likely to score positively on the tanning-modified CAGE criteria.[6]

Indoor tanning behavior among college-aged women demonstrates four distinct patterns of use: special event, spontaneous or mood, mixed, and regular year-round tanners. Cluster analysis has found statistically and clinically significant differences in tanning attitudes, intentions, behaviors, and dependence among these four groups.[18] Regular year-round tanners accounted for approximately 12% of the sample and individuals in this group initiated tanning at the earliest age, tan at the highest frequency, report the most strongly positive attitudes toward tanning, and demonstrate the highest degree of dependence.[18] Such findings are consistent with other models of addiction and dependence and suggest that psychologic dependence or an ultraviolet SRD may influence tanning behavior.

TRIALS EXAMINING BEHAVIORAL RESPONSES TO ULTRAVIOLET LIGHT

Psychologic dependence is suggested by tanners' reports of relaxation and positive mood effects as a result of ultraviolet light exposure.[6] A recent double-blind controlled study investigated whether frequent tanners demonstrate a physiologic affinity for ultraviolet light over nonultraviolet light. Frequent tanners were able to distinguish between ultraviolet and nonultraviolet light and chose to receive additional ultraviolet light over nonultraviolet light 95% of the time.[20] Thus, ultraviolet light acts as a reinforcing stimulus in frequent indoor tanners.

Ultraviolet light–induced production of cutaneous endorphins occurs in vitro and is a proposed mechanism for the reinforcing properties associated with ultraviolet light exposure. The demonstration of withdrawal symptoms in frequent tanners in response to naltrexone, an opioid antagonist, is believed to support this hypothesis.[13] The proposed mechanism is as follows. Exposure to ultraviolet radiation activates tumor suppressor protein p53 to stimulate transcription of pro-opiomelanocortin.[21] This leads to increased levels of pro-opiomelanocortin products, including β-endorphin.[20] Studies have not been able to fully substantiate this hypothesis, however.[22–24]

Whether or not tanning creates physiologic dependence was investigated by another study examining the effect of naltrexone on the preference for ultraviolet light in frequent tanners. This intervention resulted in diminished preference for ultraviolet light and the development of withdrawal symptoms in frequent tanners.[13] Other studies suggest that ultraviolet light tanning relieves pain, suggesting another possible reason for dependence.[25]

SUMMARY

Tanning is a major public health problem that is facilitated by the media, societal values, personal preference, and a possible addictive component. Tanning also is a productive area of behavioral research, spanning survey research and ultraviolet exposure studies that complement basic science studies of ultraviolet effects on cells and genes. The behavioral studies are critical, because ultraviolet exposure interventions involving ultraviolet education and awareness have not proved fruitful in reducing tanning behavior. Understanding the addictive component of ultraviolet light exposure—and the interaction of that component with other psychosocial issues—is essential for making headway in reducing excessive ultraviolet light exposure behavior.

REFERENCES

1. Zeller S, Lazovich D, Forester J, et al. Do adolescent tanners exhibit dependency? J Am Acad Dermatol 2006;54:589–96.

2. MacNeal RJ, Dinulos JG. Update on sun protection and tanning in children. Curr Opin Pediatr 2007;19: 425–9.

3. Swerdlow AJ, Weinstock MA. Do tanning lamps cause melanoma? An epidemiologic assessment. J Am Acad Dermatol 1998;38:89–98.

4. Council of Scientific Affairs. Harmful effects of ultraviolet radiation. JAMA 1989;262:380–4.

5. Knight JM, Kirincich AN, Farmer ER, et al. Awareness of the risks of tanning lamps does not influence behavior among college students. Arch Dermatol 2002;138:1311–5.

6. Poorsattar SP, Hornung RL. UV light abuse and high-risk tanning behavior among undergraduate college students. J Am Acad Dermatol 2007;56:375–9.

7. Robinson JK, Kim J, Rosenbaum S, et al. Indoor tanning knowledge, attitudes, and behavior among young adults from 1988-2007. Arch Dermatol 2008; 144(4):484–8.

8. O'Riordan DL, Field AE, Geller AC, et al. Frequent tanning bed use, weight concerns, and other health risk behaviors in adolescent females (United States). Cancer Causes Control 2006;17(5):679–86.

9. Heckman CJ, Coups EJ, Manne SL. Prevalence and correlates of indoor tanning among US adults. J Am Acad Dermatol 2008;58(5):769–80.

10. Ezzedine K, Malvy D, Mauger E, et al. Artificial and natural ultraviolet radiation exposure: beliefs and behaviour of 7200 French adults. J Eur Acad Dermatol Venereol 2008;22(2):186–94.

11. American Psychiatric Association, Task Force on DSM-IV. DSM-IV-TR: Diagnostic and statistical manual of mental disorders. Washington, DC: American Psychiatric Publishing; 2000.

12. Golan DE, Tashjian AH, Armstrong EJ, et al. Principles of pharmacology: the pathophysiologic basis of drug therapy. Baltimore: Lippincott Williams & Wilkins; 2005.

13. Kaur M, Liguori A, Land W, et al. Induction of withdrawal-like symptoms in a small randomized, controlled trial opioid blockage in frequent tanners. J Am Acad Dermatol 2006;54:709–11.

14. Sadock BJ. Kaplan and Sadock's synopsis of psychiatry. Kaplan & Sadock's synopsis of psychiatry: behavioral sciences/clinical psychiatry. Philadelphia: Lippincott Williams & Wilkins; 2003.

15. Donovan DM, Dennis M. Assessment of addictive behaviors. New York: Guilford Press; 2005.

16. Ewing JA. Detecting alcoholism. The CAGE questionnaire. JAMA 1984;252:1905–7.

17. Brandon TH, Herzog TA, Irvin JE, et al. Cognitive and social learning models of drug dependence: implications for the assessment of tobacco dependence in adolescents. Addiction 2004;99(Suppl 1): 51–77.

18. Hillhouse J, Turrisi R, Shields AL. Patterns of indoor tanning use: implications for clinical interventions. Arch Dermatol 2007;143(12):1530–5.

19. Warthan MM, Ichida T, Wagner RF Jr. UV light tanning as a type of substance-related disorder. Arch Dermatol 2005;141:963–6.

20. Feldman SR, Liguori A, Kucenic M, et al. Ultraviolet exposure is a reinforcing stimulus in frequent indoor tanners. J Am Acad Dermatol 2004;51: 45–51.

21. Cui R, Widlund HR, Feige E, et al. Central role of p53 in the suntan response and pathologic hyperpigmentation. Cell 2007;128(5):853–64.

22. Kaur M, Liguori A, Fleischer AB Jr, et al. Plasma beta-endorphin levels in frequent and infrequent tanners before and after ultraviolet and non-ultraviolet stimuli. J Am Acad Dermatol 2006;54: 919–20.

23. Wintzen M, Ostijn DM, Polderman MC, et al. Total body exposure to ultraviolet radiation does not influence plasma levels of immunoreactive beta-endorphin in man. Photodermatol Photoimmunol Photomed 2001;17:256–60.

24. Gambichler T, Bader A, Vojvodic M, et al. Plasma levels of opioid peptides after sunbed exposures. Br J Dermatol 2002;147:1207–11.

25. Kaur M, Feldman SR, Liguori A, et al. Indoor tanning relieves pain. Photodermatol Photoimmunol Photomed 2005;21:278.

Dermatologic Medication Adherence

Bridgit V. Nolan, BA[a], Steven R. Feldman, MD, PhD[b],*

KEYWORDS

- Adherence • Topical • Treatment
- Health services research

The external distribution of the skin makes it easily accessible to topical treatment. However, poor adherence to treatment regimens—in part because of a lack of adequate patient understanding, discomfort caused by certain products, undesirable cosmetic effects, or fear of long-term side effects—is frequently a major hurdle to success. Another factor limiting adherence is patients' unrealistic treatment expectations as to the rapidity of improvement or reaching full resolution of the disease. Research into treatment adherence has just begun but is already making an impact on the understanding of the mechanism of skin diseases and the response to long-term treatment. Poor outcomes in patients with other diseases states, such as hypertension and diabetes mellitus, are often due to poor adherence. In this review, the authors explore treatment adherence behavior, one of the more active areas of behavioral research in dermatology.

ADHERENCE BEHAVIOR

The term "adherence" refers to the extent to which a patient's behavior corresponds with treatment recommendations from a health care provider.[1] In the context of chronic dermatologic disease, adherence can take a variety of forms, including the avoidance of certain environmental stimuli, the consistent application of topical medications, and the initiation of lifestyle modifications, such as minimizing recreational exposure to ultraviolet light and food allergens. For most chronic diseases,

treatment does not result in a cure, but is aimed at decreasing the frequency and severity of exacerbations or slowing progression of the disease.

Treatment in dermatology differs from other specialties of medicine in that the external distribution of the skin makes it easily accessible for a variety of different treatment modalities. Topically applied preparations offer the advantages of decreased systemic side effects and direct application of potent medications to the target organ with minimal risk for systemic toxicity. However, topical therapy is also prone to error because proper application is dependent on more complex human behavior than just taking a pill. Additionally, patients frequently find treatment with topical medications to be time-consuming and unpleasant.[2,3] Poor adherence to topical therapy is ubiquitous in dermatology and has been increasingly recognized as a reason for treatment failure. Although there are treatments that work, patients do not always improve, and it has frequently been assumed that patients were using the prescribed treatments appropriately when in fact they were not. Treatment outcomes can be improved by research to better understand and improve adherence behavior. Medical resources may be better directed at encouraging patients to use treatments already available than toward developing new techniques and medications. Frequently, a skin disease can be cleared up with the appropriate use of current medications without having to resort to more risky, complicated, or costly treatment regimens.

The Center for Dermatology Research is supported by an unrestricted educational grant from Galderma Laboratories, L.P.

[a] SUNY Upstate Medical University, Weiskotten Hall, 766 Irving Avenue, Syracuse, NY 13210, USA
[b] Center for Dermatology Research, Wake Forest University School of Medicine, Medical Center Boulevard, Winston-Salem, NC 27157-1071, USA
* Corresponding author.
E-mail address: sfeldman@wfubmc.edu (S.R. Feldman).

Dermatol Clin 27 (2009) 113–120
doi:10.1016/j.det.2008.11.006

derm.theclinics.com

Medication adherence behavior, which is further divided into primary (filling prescriptions) and secondary (appropriately using medications), is of particular interest. Adherence to topical regimens is multifactorial. Patients are more likely to fill prescriptions for systemic treatments compared with topical treatments.[1] The reason for this finding is unclear—it may relate to an inherent patient belief that a pill is needed to cure, or it may result from the inconvenience and hassle associated with the long-term use of topical treatments. A recent study of dermatology patients presenting to an outpatient clinic demonstrated a 31% rate of primary nonadherence, and among the population studied, patients with psoriasis were the least adherent, with a primary nonadherence rate of nearly 50%.[1] The reasons for failure of primary adherence are not well defined but may include financial considerations, rational decisions to not use a medication because of concern about real side effects, or prior failure with similar agents. The extent of primary nonadherence behavior alone represents a significant barrier to optimal clinical outcomes in dermatologic treatment.

There are a variety of difficulties related to secondary adherence behaviors such that even when prescriptions are filled they may not be appropriately used.[4,5] Proper use of topical treatments is challenging even for individuals without significant disease burden. Inadequate patient education about the disease process and its treatment may lead to treatment errors (including overuse, underuse, and inappropriate use), thus decreasing effectiveness and increasing the potential for side effects.[6] Fear of undesirable cosmetic effects, especially with ointment-based vehicles, and real or imagined adverse side effects represent other important factors leading to poor adherence to topical treatments.[6]

Much can be done to improve patients' adherence behavior. In his review, "The importance of medication adherence in improving chronic-disease related outcomes," Dr. Raj Balkrishnan discusses a variety of approaches that can be used, including educational and behavioral strategies. These can include reminder systems and letting patients know about the importance of using their medication. Choosing treatments based on specific patients' lifestyles and personal preferences, particularly simplifying treatment regimens, is another approach.[7]

HEALTH BELIEF MODEL OF ADHERENCE BEHAVIOR

Health behavior models have been developed to define the factors affecting adherence to health recommendations. These models provide an understanding of health-related decision making and behavior and help to identify possible interventions aimed at increasing adherence behavior.[8] The health belief model is a widely used model that suggests that an individual will carry out recommended health behavior when the perceived benefits outweigh the perceived costs.[9] This model identifies four distinct contributing factors: the patient's perceived susceptibility to a condition, the perceived severity of the condition if the patient were to develop it, the perceived benefits as to the magnitude of the reduction of risk for developing a condition if a particular recommendation is followed, and the perceived costs associated with following a recommendation.[9] For example, if a patient has a parent with severe psoriasis and he develops initial lesions, he may be more likely to adhere to a treatment regimen because of the perceived susceptibility to that condition. Additionally, the perceived benefit of avoiding severe disease may outweigh any cost associated with treatment.

The health care delivery model identifies self-efficacy and external factors and their influence on an individual's health behavior. Emphasis is placed on factors related to the social, political, and economic environment in which the patient lives and to the health care structure and delivery system.[10] Social factors might include how the patient perceives the use of topical medications will be received or responded to by a spouse or significant other, by family members, by those in his work or social environment, and perhaps even by casual contacts, such as people on the street or in the supermarket. If a negative response is expected, this situation can be intimidating and inhibiting. As an example, in the first several months of treatment, patients who are using isotretinoin frequently experience worsening acne, redness of the face, extreme dryness and peeling, and cracking of the lips. These side effects may be viewed as socially unacceptable in our appearance-obsessed culture. Economic factors certainly play a huge role in patient adherence. Patients on a tight budget may choose to spend their money on other, more necessary items. Many people who need things such as a new pair of glasses to see, gasoline for their car, or diabetes medicine to keep their blood sugar under control may elect to purchase these items rather than acne medication. Some teenagers might even chose to spend their money on frivolous but more enjoyable items, such as cosmetics, cigarettes, alcohol, entertainment, or clothing.

Social cognitive theory uses the term "reciprocal determinism" to describe the complex, continuous, and multidirectional interaction between the individual, his environment, and his behavior.[11] These interactions are important in understanding adherence behavior because outcomes of treatment influence patient satisfaction and future adherence behavior.[12] There are two sides to this causal relationship: for some, better outcomes may increase perceived benefit of treatment, thus resulting in greater future adherence to topical medication; for others, clinical improvement may decrease patients' adherence by reducing the perceived need for continual treatment (and potentially reducing adverse effects of long-term treatment exposures).

STUDIES EXAMINING ADHERENCE BEHAVIOR IN DERMATOLOGY

In this section, the authors examine the adherence behavior of patients with psoriasis, acne, and atopic dermatitis.

Psoriasis

Psoriasis is a chronic disease associated with significant distress and impairment. The chronicity and incurability of disease, the availability of effective treatments, and the need for long-term application renders psoriasis an ideal candidate for the study of adherence to topical treatments. Consequently, psoriasis has been a topic of much research related to adherence rates, factors influencing adherence rates, the most effective and/or preferred vehicle for treatment, and reasons for treatment failure.

The first line of treatment for mild to moderate disease is topical corticosteroids.[13,14] Treatment adherence is generally poor, and in some studies patients with psoriasis have ranked among the most nonadherent.[1] Estimates of nonadherence rates among patients with psoriasis range between 30% and 50%.[1,6] There are a variety of factors believed to influence adherence to treatment regimens in patients with psoriasis, including concerns about medication side effects, unpleasant cosmetic effects, the inconvenient and time-consuming aspect of applications, and inadequate education of the patient as to the chronicity of the disease; these factors ultimately lead to patient frustration.

A recent evaluation of psoriasis patients used a self-administered questionnaire to identify motivating factors for failure to adhere to topical corticosteroid treatment. More than one-third of the patients admitted nonadherence to the treatment regimen, thus confirming the results of prior studies on psoriasis.[1,6] The major reasons for deviation from the prescribed treatment regimen were dissatisfaction related to medication efficacy expectation, fear of adverse side effects, and inconvenience.[6] These findings are consistent with the health belief model, which states that an individual will adhere to a treatment regimen when perceived benefits outweigh perceived costs. In another study on psoriasis, the top two reasons for nonadherence to therapy were being busy (25%) and being fed up (21%).[15] Both adherent and nonadherent patients expressed concerns related to topical medication safety, suggesting a need for better patient education.[6] Recent research also suggests a temporal relationship between office visits and adherence rates, with patients exhibiting better adherence behavior closer to the time of office visits. Therefore, an immediate follow-up visit after the initiation of treatment in addition to frequent follow-up visits may be effective in increasing adherence and improving clinical outcomes.[6]

Psychologic factors related to acceptance of chronic illness may also modulate adherence behavior. Lack of or incomplete acceptance leads to lower adherence, delayed improvement, self-medication, and psychologic distress.[16] Factors influencing the acceptance of illness include self-efficacy, optimism, and health locus of control (one's conviction that one's health depends on oneself or others). The presence of depression, denial, and distress complicate and in some cases diminish adherence and successful treatment outcome.[17-19] These findings identify possible areas for interventions to improve acceptance of an illness and improve clinical outcome.

Acne Vulgaris

Acne is a common dermatologic condition affecting adolescents, teenagers, and adults. The clinical course and severity of acne are highly variable, and although a linear relationship does not exist between clinical severity and quality of life, depression, lowered self-esteem, and poor interpersonal relationships are reported by many patients with acne. Although there are a variety of treatments for acne with well-established clinical efficacy, adherence to these regimens is often poor. Studies show that adherence to treatment is associated with lower measures of disease severity in patients with mild to moderate acne.[20] Adolescents have been consistently identified as being at high risk for nonadherent behavior, and in one study the estimate of adherence to acne treatment regimens among college students was 12.5%.[21] Other studies show that nearly 20% of patients with acne fail to return for follow-up visits and that by three months less than half of patients adhere.[22,23]

One of the primary barriers to successful adherence to acne regimens in adolescents and teenagers is the nature of acne and the treatments available. Most acne treatments require long-term adherence to achieve resolution.[24] Medications that fail to produce appreciable improvement within a brief period of time are associated with a decreased adherence.[25] Inadequate patient education allows for unrealistic expectations. Patients' expectation as to the speed of improvement is considerably faster than the actual time needed to achieve improvement in acne.[22,26,27] Additionally, continued maintenance of treatment is required to suppress future breakouts. For treatment to be effective, patients must have a basic understanding of the course of disease.

Patients may not accept the fact that long-term benefits outweigh short-term discomfort. Side effects from topical acne treatments include irritation, burning, itching, a red face, and staining of clothing. Additionally, for female patients who wish to wear makeup and other skin care products, applying multiple topical medications may be undesirable because they may change the appearance of makeup such as foundation, bronzer, and blush.[24] For teenagers, this type of treatment may be particularly difficult because they have limited experience with long-term medical adherence, have difficulty delaying gratification, and are easily frustrated.[24] Treatment regimen factors also play a role; specifically, as dosing frequency and number of medications increases, adherence decreases.

A variety of psychosocial factors affect treatment adherence in patients with acne. One recent study demonstrates a significant negative correlation between scores on the Dermatology Life Quality Index and adherence behavior.[28] The major factors associated with nonadherent behavior in this study were being "fed up," "forgetful," or "too busy."[28] The use of quality-of-life scales, particularly in teenage patients with acne, may increase detection of high-impact disease and patients who need special attention for improved adherence behavior.[29]

Interventions to improve adherence behavior in the treatment of patients with acne have focused on strengthening the doctor-patient relationship, simplifying treatment regimens, and understanding patient preferences and values and their incorporation into the treatment plan. Patients should also be educated on expected treatment outcomes to avoid frustration. There are additional recommendations for dealing with teenagers, who constitute a major proportion of patients seeking treatment for acne and who are the least likely to be adherent. It is important to take into account teenagers' school activities, sports, personal schedules, and in women, the preference for using makeup.

Atopic Dermatitis

Atopic dermatitis is a common skin disorder with clinical manifestations varying with age. Often three stages can be identified—in infancy, in childhood, and in adolescence and adulthood.[30] In each stage, pruritus is the most important and persistent symptom and frequently impairs the patient's quality of life.[30] More than 50% of children who are affected in the first two years of life do not have signs of IgE sensitization, but they do become sensitized during the course of atopic dermatitis.[30] Because the disease begins in infancy and effective treatment may help to decrease later sensitization to environmental allergens, promoting adherence and motivation on the part of the primary caregiver is important.

Treatment relies on topical corticosteroids and immunomodulators. However, a recent study of children with atopic dermatitis demonstrated that adherence to a simple, static treatment regimen consisting of application of triamcinolone cream was only 32% over an eight-week period.[31] Other studies demonstrate that self-reported adherence to topical corticosteroid treatment is greater than objectively measured adherence and that adherence decreases as the length of time from initiation of medication increases.[32]

Poor adherence behavior should be considered when patients with atopic dermatitis are not responding to topical corticosteroid treatment. Studies of patients with atopic dermatitis have revealed low levels of adherence but have offered little in the way of evidence-based recommendations for improvement. Barriers to adherence are numerous and may include caregiver fatigue, confusion as to the treatment plan, and fear of adverse side effects. The fear of side effects associated with topical corticosteroid use is a potent factor motivating treatment nonadherence in patients with atopic dermatitis. In a recent study of patients with atopic dermatitis, 72% reported concern about side effects of topical corticosteroid use, particularly skin atrophy, and 24% reported nonadherence as a result of these fears.[33] There is significant variation among dermatologists in the perceived safety and potential for side-effects of topical corticosteroid preparations.[34] Inaccurate assessment of safety can lead to inappropriate treatment decisions on the part of physicians. An inadequate level of patient education and understanding increases fear surrounding topical corticosteroid use, ultimately resulting in decreased adherence.[35] Efforts to better educate patients, their parents, and health care workers are essential to improve clinical outcomes in patients with atopic dermatitis.

Until options based in behavior research become available, common sense may be the best guide to improving adherence behavior in patients with atopic dermatitis. The treatment regimen should be made as simple as possible and explained verbally and in writing. Patient education on treatment with topical corticosteroids should include their potency and frequency, application sites, quantity, and duration of application. Additionally, differentiation between therapies to be used for maintenance and exacerbation must be communicated to ensure appropriate use and to minimize side effects. Demonstration of treatment application and parental education has also been recommended.[35]

Numerous studies have demonstrated significant concern related to side effects of corticosteroid therapy, and in some cases these concerns have been associated with nonadherent behavior.[33] Many of the side effects of corticosteroids are only a problem with long-term use, yet concerns about side effects may still limit patients' initial use of treatment. Postponing the discussion of potential long-term side effects until after a short-term improvement has occurred has been suggested as a means to promote medication adherence.[31] Additionally, a strong doctor-patient relationship may alleviate some of the anxiety associated with topical corticosteroid use.[36]

Parallels in pathophysiologic mechanisms, clinical courses, and treatment plans between asthma and atopic dermatitis may provide insight into methods for increasing patient adherence. Both are chronic inflammatory conditions characterized by waxing and waning symptomatology that at times require complex treatment regimen. Some studies have suggested that increased patient and caregiver education, the use of written action plans (WAPs), and other follow-up devices may be helpful among asthma patients.[37,38]

STUDIES TO IMPROVE ADHERENCE

Efforts to improve patients' adherence to treatment regimens could have a profound impact on dermatologic disease and patients' quality of life. Several factors are believed to affect patient adherence, including the doctor-patient relationship, treatment regimen factors, patient education, and psychosocial factors.

Doctor-Patient Relationship

The establishment of an effective doctor-patient relationship, characterized by good communication, trust, and caring, is consistently identified as the most important factor influencing patient adherence.[36,39,40] Approximately 70% of adherent patients follow the treatment regimen because they view their physician as a caring advisor and trust his instructions.[41] Good communication between doctor and patient and involvement of the patient in planning the treatment regimen are important aspects of the doctor-patient relationship.[42] Respecting patient preferences, especially with regard to vehicle selection, is often overlooked but is essential to establishing a treatment plan to which a patient will adhere.[24] Additionally, anticipating impediments and resolving adherence issues requires an understanding of the patient's economic, social, and cultural context. Physicians need to have a kind, empathetic nature and to be flexible in altering treatment plans to better accommodate patient preference.[24] At all times, it is important for the physician to avoid being judgmental and to encourage discussion.[24]

Respect for Patient Preferences and Lifestyle Factors

Patients prefer treatment regimens that are simple, not messy, and easily integrated into their personal routine. The extent to which the treatment regimen is compatible with the patient's preferences and lifestyle strongly influences patient adherence. Patients with psoriasis tend to prefer non–ointment-based preparations, despite the commonly held belief that ointment-based preparations are most effective.[43] Medications delivered in vehicles that patients prefer are more likely to be used.[44] Patient preference for one agent over another and the willingness to use it likely affects therapeutic outcome more than any difference in efficacy between agents does. Additionally, simplifying the treatment plan, whether through reduction of the number of agents used or the frequency of dosage, promotes adherence.[45] Because many dermatologic conditions are chronic and require long-term management, it is essential to take into account patient preferences when planning a treatment regimen.

Patient and Caregiver Education

Improved patient and caregiver education is important in facilitating rational decision making and adherence behavior. The physician should explain the pathogenesis of the condition in simple language because this knowledge fosters understanding of the rationale for treatment. For patients with other chronic disease states, such as asthma, educational efforts resulted in increased adherence and better clinical outcomes.[39] Education about treatment should include elements of patient instruction on proper technique and realistic outcome expectations. Instructions on how to take or appropriately apply medications should be provided in a simple, clear manner, both verbally and in written form.

Parallels in disease mechanisms and progression between asthma and atopic dermatitis suggest that the same interventions may work for both diseases. The use of WAPs increases adherence among pediatric asthma patients, with a resulting decrease in asthma exacerbations and an improvement in health outcomes.[46,47] WAPs function as a communication aid between the patient (or the patient's parent) and the physician, clarifying potentially confusing aspects of the treatment regimen. WAPs promote adherence by providing a visual stimulus to remind the patient to follow the treatment schedule, and such visual cues lead to increased adherence in asthmatic patients.[48] WAPs may also improve the patients' understanding of treatment goals (e.g., differentiating management versus cure), leading to realistic treatment expectations and decreasing frustrations associated with perceived treatment failure.[46] Additionally, WAPs are associated with positive patient perceptions, and this may have an effect on treatment adherence independent of the educational value of the intervention.[49] The similarities between asthma and atopic dermatitis (specifically the chronicity of the disease, the complexity of treatment regimens, the pervasive low levels of adherence to treatment, and the need for caregiver involvement) suggest that the use of WAPs may represent a helpful intervention in increasing adherence to treatment in patients with atopic dermatitis. To date, there are no studies assessing the efficacy of WAPs in pediatric patients with atopic dermatitis, although this is an area that is worthy of further investigation.

Psychosocial Factors

Chronic disease states pose a unique challenge for patients and their physicians. The long duration, exacerbations, recurrences, and ultimate incurability of the disease may lead to patient frustration. Significant distress due to restrictions imposed by the disease or its treatment regime decreases quality of life for those afflicted. Studies have shown that adherence rates for people with chronic disease are significantly lower than adherence rates for people with acute disease and that

these rates further decrease after 6 months of therapy.[24] Adjustment to chronic disease is a complex process that is modified by a variety of internal and external factors.[16] Optimism, positive coping mechanisms, and acceptance of illness are associated with increased adherence. Possible interventions to increase adherence in patients with chronic dermatologic conditions might include cognitive behavioral therapy techniques such as thought monitoring and thought blocking, distraction, and relaxation.[16] Future studies into the efficacy of such interventions will be necessary to determine if they are truly effective.

SUMMARY

Behavior research in dermatology has given recent insight into major dermatologic issues. These studies highlight the multiplicity of factors involved in adherence behavior and may lead to a better understanding of why patients respond or don't respond to treatment. These studies are also changing how we view what we do today and offer suggestions as to how we can do things better.

The knowledge gained from behavioral research impacts the care of patients immediately and profoundly. Success in the treatment of dermatologic disease is directly related to the degree of adherence, and the potential for improving patients' lives right now by tailoring treatment to their needs and thus increasing adherence is enormous.

REFERENCES

1. Storm A, Andersen SE, Benfeldt E, et al. One in 3 prescriptions are never redeemed: primary nonadherence in an outpatient clinic. J Am Acad Dermatol 2008;59(1):27–33.
2. Richards HL, Fortune DG, O'Sullivan TM, et al. Patients with psoriasis and their compliance with medication. J Am Acad Dermatol 1999;41:581–3.
3. Rapp SR, Exum ML, Reboussin DM, et al. The physical, psychological and social impact of psoriasis. J Health Psychol 1997;2:525–37.
4. Ulff E, Maroti M, Kettis-Lindblad A, et al. Single application of a fluorescent test cream by healthy volunteers: assessment of treated and neglected body sites. Br J Dermatol 2007;156:974–8.
5. Savary J, Ortonne JP, Aractingi S. The right dose in the right place: an overview of current prescription, instruction and application modalities for topical psoriasis treatments. J Eur Acad Dermatol Venereol 2005;19(Suppl 3):14–7.
6. Brown KK, Rehmus WE, Kimball AB. Determining the relative importance of patient motivations for

nonadherence to topical corticosteroid therapy in psoriasis. J Am Acad Dermatol 2006;55(4):207–13.

7. Balkrishnan R. The importance of medication adherence in improving chronic-disease related outcomes: what we know and what we need to further know. Med Care 2005;43(6):517–20.

8. Redding CA, Rossi JS, Rossi SR, et al. Health behavior models. The International Electronic Journal of Health Education 2000;3:180–93.

9. Janz NK, Becker MH. The health belief model: a decade later. Health Educ Q 1984;11(1):1–47.

10. Aday LA, Andersen R. A framework for the study of access to medical care. Health Serv Res 1974;9(3): 208–20.

11. Bandura A. Social foundations of thought and action: a social cognitive theory. Englewood Cliffs (NJ): Prentice-Hall; 1986.

12. Feldman SR, Horn EJ, Balkrishnan R, et al, for the International Psoriasis Council. Psoriasis: improving adherence to topical therapy. J Am Acad Dermatol 2008 Oct 1 [Epub ahead of print].

13. Lebwohl M, Ali S. Treatment of psoriasis. Part 1. Topical therapy and phototherapy. J Am Acad Dermatol 2001;45:487–98.

14. Habif T. Psoriasis and other papulosquamous diseases. Clinical dermatology: a color guide to diagnosis and therapy. 4th edition. New York: Mosby Inc.; 2004. p. 209–25.

15. Gokdemir G, Ari S, Köşlü A. Adherence to treatment in patients with psoriasis vulgaris: Turkish experience. J Eur Acad Dermatol Venereol 2008;22(3): 330–5.

16. Zalewska A, Miniszewska J, Chodkiewicz J, et al. Acceptance of chronic illness in psoriasis vulgaris patients. J Eur Acad Dermatol Venereol 2007;21(2): 235–42.

17. Kulkarni AS, Balkrishnan R, Camacho FT, et al. Medication and health care service utilization related to depressive symptoms in older adults with psoriasis. J Drugs Dermatol 2004;3(6):661–6.

18. Awadalla FC, Yentzer B, Balkrishnan R, et al. A role for denial in poor adherence to psoriasis treatment. J Dermatolog Treat 2007;18(6):324–5.

19. Awadalla FC, Balkrishnan R, Feldman SR. The distress of psoriasis doesn't necessarily imply good treatment adherence: a lesson from the treatment of sexually transmitted disease. J Dermatolog Treat 2008;19(3):132–3.

20. Jones-Caballero M, Pedrosa E, Peñas PF. Self-reported adherence to treatment and quality of life in mild to moderate acne. Dermatology 2008;217(4): 309–14.

21. Parsons R, Wright N, Wilson L. Evaluation of patients' compliance with medical practitioners' prescriptions: university health center experience. J Am Coll Health Assoc 1980;28:342–5.

22. McEvoy B, Nydegger R, Williams G. Factors related to patient compliance in the treatment of acne vulgaris. Int J Dermatol 2003;42:274–80.

23. Flanders PA, McNamara JR. Enhancing acne medication compliance: a comparison of strategies. Behav Res Ther 1985;23:225–7.

24. Baldwin HE. Tricks for improving compliance with acne therapy. Dermatol Ther 2006;19(4):224–36.

25. Denzii C. Medication noncompliance: what is the problem? Manag Care 2000;9:7–12.

26. Rasmussen J, Smith S. Patient concepts and misconceptions about acne. Arch Dermatol 1983; 119:570–2.

27. Tan J, Vasey K, Fung K. Beliefs and perceptions of patients with acne. J Am Acad Dermatol 2001;44: 439–45.

28. Zaghloul SS, Cunliffe WJ, Goodfield MJ. Objective assessment of compliance with treatments in acne. Br J Dermatol 2005;152(5):1015–21.

29. Dréno B. Assessing quality of life in patients with acne vulgaris: implications for treatment. Am J Clin Dermatol 2006;7(2):99–106.

30. Bieber T. Mechanisms of disease: atopic dermatitis. N Engl J Med 2008;358(14):1483–94.

31. Krejci-Manwaring J, Tusa MG, Carroll C, et al. Stealth monitoring of adherence to topical medication: adherence is very poor in children with atopic dermatitis. J Am Acad Dermatol 2007;56(2):211–6.

32. Conde JF, Kaur M, Fleischer AM Jr, et al. Adherence to clocortolone pivalate cream 0.1% in a pediatric population with atopic dermatitis. Cutis 2008;81(5):435–41.

33. Charman CR, Morris AD, Williams HC. Topical corticosteroid phobia in patients with atopic eczema. Br J Dermatol 2000;142:931–6.

34. Charman CR, Williams HC. Dermatologists' perceived safety of topical corticosteroids in children with atopic eczema [abstract]. Br J Dermatol 2001; 145:127.

35. Beattie PE, Lewis-Jones MS. Parental knowledge of topical therapies in the treatment of childhood atopic dermatitis. Clin Exp Dermatol 2003;28(5):549–53.

36. Ohya Y, Williams H, Steptoe A, et al. Psychosocial factors and adherence to treatment advice in childhood atopic dermatitis. J Invest Dermatol 2001; 117(4):852–7.

37. Bhogal S, Zemek R, Ducharme FM. Written action plans for asthma in children. Cochrane Database Syst Rev 2006;(3):CD005306.

38. Cabana MD, Rand CS, Wu AW, et al. Why don't patients follow clinical practice guidelines? A framework for improvement. JAMA 1999;282:1458–65.

39. Fish JE, Lung CL. Adherence to asthma therapy. Ann Allergy Asthma Immunol 2001;86:24–30.

40. Bender BG. Overcoming barriers to nonadherence in asthma treatment. J Allergy Clin Immunol 2002; 109:S554–9.

41. Felkey B. Adherence screening and monitoring. Am Pharm 1995;NS35:42–51.

42. Gillisen A. Patient's adherence in asthma. J Physiol Pharmacol 2007;58(Suppl 5(Pt 1)):205–22.

43. Warino L, Balkrishnan R, Feldman SR. Clobetasol proprionate for psoriasis: are ointments really more potent? J Drugs Dermatol 2006;5(6):527–32.

44. Gottlieb A, Ford R, Spellman M. The efficacy and tolerability of clobetasol propionate foam 0.05% in the treatment of mild to moderate plaque-type psoriasis of nonscalp region. J Cutan Med Surg 2003;7:185–92.

45. Eisen SA, Miller DK, Woodward RS, et al. The effect of prescribed daily dose frequency on patient medication compliance. Arch Intern Med 1990;150:1881–4.

46. Chisolm SS, Taylor SL, Balkrishnan R, et al. Written action plans: potential for improving outcomes in children with atopic dermatitis. J Am Acad Dermatol 2008 May 28 [Epub ahead of print].

47. Boychuk RB, Demesa CJ, Kiyabu KM, et al. Change in approach and delivery of medical care in children with asthma: results from a multicenter emergency department educational asthma management program. Pediatrics 2006;117:S145–51.

48. Ruoff G. Effects of flow sheet implementation on physician performance in the management of asthmatic patients. Fam Med 2002;34:514–7.

49. Douglass J, Aroni R, Goeman D, et al. A qualitative study of action plans for asthma. BMJ 2002;324:1003–5.

Survey Research in Dermatology: Guidelines for Success

Adam Asarch, BA[a], Annie Chiu, MD[b], Alexa B. Kimball, MD, MPH[c,d],
Robert P. Dellavalle, MD, PhD, MSPH[e,f,g,*]

KEYWORDS

- Dermatology • Survey research • Response rate
- Questionnaire design • Reporting survey results

Public health and epidemiology depend heavily upon well-designed surveys to gather opinions, follow trends in attitudes, establish correlations, and make educated predictions. The dermatologic literature has benefited from a broad array of recent survey topics including patient and physician opinions on psoriasis,[1–10] atopic dermatitis,[11–15] bullous disease,[16,17] contact dermatitis,[18] skin cancer.[19–24] Surveys have also assessed patient satisfaction, symptoms, quality of life, disease comorbities, and opinions of trainees and the general public.[25–28] Because of their ubiquitous use, the proper design and implementation of surveys is paramount.

To optimally use surveys and limit error, a number of key factors must be addressed. Most importantly, investigators must develop a testable hypothesis that holds significance for the medical community. Once a hypothesis has been formulated, investigators must determine the target survey population to analyze. Furthermore, for a survey to provide significance, investigators should aim for acceptable response rates by a desired, target population. Many factors, which we will review in this article, can aid investigators in increasing response rates. Finally, developing valid questions with relevant response options that address the hypothesis is of the utmost importance for investigators. These basic guidelines, which can be applied to dermatologic surveys as well, will aid investigators in using surveys efficiently.

GUIDELINES FOR SURVEY RESEARCH
Basics

The same principles that guide successful survey research for the general community can be applied in the field of dermatology. The underlying goal of survey research is to estimate the characteristics of a defined population by surveying a representative sample of individuals from that population.[29,30] To accurately gain representative information, a number of key guidelines should generally be followed: (1) investigators must gain access to a large enough sample size to allow for statistically significant analysis;[29,31] (2) the group of individuals being surveyed, who possess the trait being studied, should have a known probability or

Adam Asarch and Annie Chiu contributed equally to this work.

[a] Tufts University School of Medicine, Boston, MA 02111, USA
[b] Cedars-Sinai Medical Group, 200 North Robertson Boulevard, #202, Beverly Hills, CA 90211, USA
[c] Department of Dermatology, Massachusetts General Hospital, Harvard Medical School, Boston, MA 02114, USA
[d] Clinical Unit for Research Trials in Skin (CURTIS), Massachusetts General and Brigham and Women's Hospitals, 50 Staniford Street, #246, Boston, MA 02114, USA
[e] Department of Dermatology, University of Colorado at Denver and Health Sciences Center, Denver, CO 80045, USA
[f] Dermatology Service, Department of Veterans Affairs Medical Center, 1055 Clermont Street, Mail Code 165, Denver, CO 80220, USA
[g] Colorado School of Public Health, 13001 E. 17th Place, Campus Box B119, Aurora, CO, 80045, USA
* Corresponding author. Colorado School of Public Health, 13001 E. 17th Place, Campus Box B119, Aurora, CO, 80045.
E-mail address: robert.dellavalle@ucdenver.edu (R.P. Dellavalle).

Dermatol Clin 27 (2009) 121–131
doi:10.1016/j.det.2008.11.001
0733-8635/08/$ – see front matter © 2009 Published by Elsevier Inc.

chance of being selected for the survey;[30] (3) investigators need to aim for acceptable response rates from the selected survey population;[32] and (4) questions must be developed that can address a hypothesis, provide consistently measurable and interpretable responses, and allow respondents to answer in a nonbiased fashion.[30]

To successfully complete a survey, investigators must first define the target survey population to be analyzed. This necessitates developing parameters of the survey population for study inclusion, which should be tailored to the specific goals of the study. Because the entire survey population will typically be large, researchers can survey a sample of their population to obtain the characteristics of the wider group. This is known as survey sampling.

Quantitative and nonquantitative sampling methods are available. Ideally, investigators will use quantitative methods such as random or stratified sampling. However, in certain instances random sampling can be difficult for investigators to initiate. Stratified sampling is a variant of random sampling where individuals are stratified according to a certain trait. For instance, patients may be stratified according to sex. Thus, only males or females would then be randomly selected for the survey. A third option is systematic sampling, where every nth element is randomly selected from the survey list (ie, every 50th individual on a registry would be selected for the survey). When random, stratified, and systemic sampling methods are unfeasible, researchers may resort to nonquantitative sampling such as convenience sampling and judgment sampling. Convenience sampling involves sampling individuals at a single institution or practice. This method provides obvious advantages for investigators, but can lead to significant error. Judgment sampling, as its name implies, involves using the investigator's judgment to choose a survey sample. For instance, an investigator may choose to only evaluate patients of a certain region with the pretext that this will represent the entire population.

When performing survey sampling, each person must have a known chance of being selected. If the sampling chance is known, the researcher can use weighting to construct accurate estimates from the survey. When the chance is unknown (eg, when a convenience sample is used at a single dermatology office), the only way to determine representativeness of the sample is to compare patient characteristics with the larger population that they are intended to represent. However, these comparisons cannot often be made. Regardless of sampling methods, investigators must make every attempt to evaluate the ability

of their survey sample to represent the wider survey population being evaluated.

Furthermore, investigators must have a method for obtaining access to the sample population. This is known as the sample frame. Essentially, researchers can obtain access to a population through a list frame, or an area frame. A list frame represents a list of individuals provided by a certain institution. For example, investigators could obtain a list of dermatologists from the American Academy of Dermatology. An area frame takes a geographic area and extracts a list of individuals from that area. For instance, investigators could select a list of cities, and then extract a list of dermatologists from those cities. Investigators must determine the most appropriate method for generating their list based on the constructs of their study.

Response Rates

Obtaining a high response rate should be continually stressed when performing survey research. The response rate is the proportion of individuals selected for a survey who actually reply. High response levels are necessary for limiting nonresponse error, or the error that results from differences in the responding versus the nonresponding population.[30,32–34] Asch and colleagues[35] found a mean response rate of approximately 60% for surveys published in medical journals. In general, it may be difficult to publish a report with a response rate lower than 30% to 50%. However, a survey with a low response rate can be scientifically meaningful if it can be shown that the respondents are not biased. Unfortunately, low response rates often mean that only a selective group has responded. Nonetheless, if the responding group is representative, then the data can still be meaningful.

Persistence is perhaps the most important factor in attaining high response levels. Multiple mailings or phone calls may be necessary when attempting to obtain answers.[30,36,37] Contacting participants before sending questionnaires increases responses, as does follow-up contact.[38]

Dillman[30] outlines three principles for achieving responsiveness: rewards, cost, and trust. Providing rewards in the form of financial incentives or altruistic incentives can help in enticing individuals to respond. Limiting cost to the survey population by providing return envelopes, making questions understandable, and ensuring anonymity are also important. Finally, providing credentials and explaining the survey's importance can build essential trust between investigators and the surveyed population.[30]

Incentives to increase survey completion can range widely. For instance, if a certain population is driven by the desire for practical information, investigators may offer a preliminary summary of results for participants. Not surprisingly, monetary compensation has been shown to consistently increase response rates. Monetary incentives can range from a drawing prize to an actual dollar amount. Interestingly, a recent meta-analysis of monetary incentives demonstrated that amounts larger than $5 appear to yield diminishing benefits.[39,40] A smaller reward provided up front with the survey request yields a greater response rate than a larger reward promised on completion of the survey.[30]

A number of specific techniques have been shown to increase response rates for mailed surveys. Including a pre-addressed, prestamped envelope for return of the survey is a must. Follow-up letters, accompanied with a second copy of the questionnaire, can increase response rates by 13%.[35] Additionally, university and hospital stationary can significantly augment replies by lending credibility.[41] Including a pen with the survey is another low-cost method for improving response levels. This simple, inexpensive technique may increase responses by up to 7%.[42] Dillman's[30] protocol recommends 5 points of contact to increase response rates: an advance letter, the survey, a reminder postcard, and two more survey mailings.

Always provide a realistic estimate of time required for survey completion. For mailed surveys, have this information concisely and prominently displayed on the front page. For Internet-based surveys, where subjects do not have the ability to leaf through the study, displaying the estimated completion time is important. Progress bars, which graphically demonstrate time to completion, are also effective. These simple techniques will decrease the likelihood that participants will quit mid-survey.

Types of Surveys

The most common surveys are mail and phone surveys. However, Web-based surveys are becoming more commonplace.[30] Direct patient interviews and questionnaires that are completed in person are frequently used as well.[5–7] Different methods of data collection offer their own advantages and disadvantages (**Table 1**).

The most basic method of data collection is the in-person, face-to-face interview. Subjects often find it difficult to turn down investigators in person. Furthermore, this method allows for longer surveys and detailed answers, and it provides subjects with a chance to clarify questions. Because the in-person survey can be prearranged, it is considered

less intrusive. As a result, higher response rates are often noted. In addition, the length of the survey can be greatly increased. Cost and time constraints as well as the potential for bias are disadvantages of the personal interview. The survey does not offer anonymity, and time constraints may lead to participation by individuals unrepresentative of the general population in some cases.

Telephone surveys are another major survey method. Because most people have access to telephones, the method offers the advantage of near universal coverage. Like the in-person survey, an interviewer can elicit longer, more exact answers. Respondents can also clarify a question. Another advantage of telephone surveys is that they can be conducted from a centralized location, which increases possibilities for supervision and quality control. However, the telephone survey has drawbacks. The preponderance of "telemarketing" has made is difficult to initiate legitimate scientific surveys by phone. If calls are made at a particular time of day, telephone surveys may result in selection bias. For instance, if calls are made during work hours, participants are likely to either work at home or not work. To bypass this particular problem, investigators often call in the evening, typically between 6 and 9 PM. Unfortunately, calls during this time period are often very disruptive, and investigators may note a dramatic reduction in response levels. Additionally, the increased use of cell phones, caller ID, and answering machines and services can limit an investigator's ability to obtain a good sample and high response rate.

Mailed surveys are perhaps the most commonly used method for obtaining information. Minimization of cost and assurance of anonymity make the method very attractive for investigators. The mailed survey not only allows for far-reaching access, but also allows for flexibility and independence by respondents. However, the preponderance of mail and "junk mail" can make it difficult to achieve high response rates. For mailed surveys, investigators must ensure that questions are understandable and clear. Unlike in other methods, participants will not have the option to clarify questions. A further disadvantage of mailed surveys is that investigators cannot be assured of who filled out the survey. Time remains a major drawback for the mailed survey. Even if a subject plans to respond, significant delays should be expected. Investigators must set acceptable time limits before initiating mailings.[43] A high-quality mail survey will typically take at least 6 to 8 weeks to complete the survey administration protocol.

Table 1
Survey types: advantages and disadvantages

Data Collection Method	Advantages	Disadvantages
In-person interview	• Increases response rates • Longer surveys tolerated	• Cost • Time • Not anonymous
Telephone interview	• Near universal availability • Minimizes misinterpretation of questions	• Disruptive • Selection bias of nonworking or working population depending on when call is placed • Not completely anonymous • Cell phones, caller ID, answering machines have decreased the utility of telephone surveys
Mailed Surveys	• Inexpensive • Convenient for respondent • Results anonymous	• Time to data collection can be delayed • Response rates may be lower
Internet/e-mail surveys	• Inexpensive • Data collection can be greatly expedited • Allows automated randomization of questions	• Selection bias against poorest and oldest members of population • Potential for low response rates

Web-based surveys have become one of the most rapidly growing survey methods. They offer the advantage of collecting information in a rapid, inexpensive fashion. Depending on the sophistication of the survey tool, data analysis can also be expedited. Multiple tools such as surveymonkey.com and Dillman's Tailored Design Method are available to help investigators design and disperse their Web-based surveys.[30] Unfortunately, response rates to computer-based surveys can be highly variable. Recent studies with physicians showed significantly lower response rates for Web-based surveys than for mailed surveys.[44,45] Access to the Internet may be limited for the poorest and oldest individuals in society. Researchers must be careful to screen for duplicate responses from the same subject, which can significantly bias survey results. Obtaining a list of e-mail addresses to include in the survey remains a major issue for Internet-based surveys. Encouraging people to pay attention to the e-mail request can also be difficult. Finally, investigators should also consider that most e-mail servers have automated "spam" filters that can block mass e-mails.

DESIGNING YOUR SURVEY

The primary rule for survey design is simplicity. A clear and attractive layout of a questionnaire can greatly improve response rates. Concise and simple language is a must, because technical, difficult-to-understand questions will frustrate even the most educated of survey respondents. Furthermore, difficult-to-understand questions will not elicit valid responses.

Survey Format

The creation of a concise, aesthetically pleasing survey will greatly aid investigators in obtaining a high response. Start with a short message that provides the credentials of the investigators, as well as the general objectives and estimated time commitment of the study. The questionnaire should be at least 12-point font with adequate spacing and margins to allow for easy readability. For computer-based surveys, minimize distracting graphics and brightly colored backgrounds, and fit text within typical monitor sizes. Participants find horizontal scrolling both annoying and confusing. Answer choices should be placed at a location where the eye naturally tracks, typically in a straight line down the left side of the page with one answer per line. Participants prefer vertically oriented answer choices and bolding of questions and directions. For Web-based surveys, click-tabs are more "user friendly" than drop-down/pull-down menus. Clearly spaced answer choices can also ease the process of data tabulation for investigators.

Opening with easier, interesting questions that are central to the topic of the survey may increase the likelihood that the respondent will continue. Grouping related questions can make a survey easier to complete, but may increase the likelihood that subjects will choose the same answer without thinking. Be aware of unwanted redundancy or questions that do not directly address the established hypothesis, as they can add unnecessary length and time to a survey and result in decreased response rate.

An investigator should be aware and attempt to avoid biases that may be built into a particular survey design. When a long list of answer choices are presented for a question, subjects tend to choose answers that appear earlier on the list. This is particularly true for pull-down/drop-down menus on computerized surveys. Alphabetized lists can help address this problem by allowing respondents to go straight to an answer, but this assumes that respondents have an answer in mind. All answers provided on a survey should have equal ease of visibility. Aligning answers along the same part of the page can be helpful in accomplishing this goal. Subjects will choose only from the choices seen, and survey designers should try to ensure no page breaks in a middle of an answer choice set.

Survey Questions

The three most common types of survey questions are multiple choice, numeric open-ended, and text open-ended (**Fig. 1**). Although useful for gathering opinions and information, text open-ended questions yield less response because of the effort required. These questions are also difficult for respondents to answer. As a result, investigators typically use multiple-choice or numeric open-ended types of questions (see **Fig. 1**). When designing questions, issues of validity and reliability should also be considered. Validity evaluates whether the question is eliciting the information sought by the researcher, whereas reliability evaluates whether the question will elicit the same answer if asked again. Reliability should be addressed by asking the same question in multiple ways. Validity should be addressed by using clear language with straightforward meaning.

To capture opinions and attitudes, a commonly used tool is either the 4-point or 5-point Likert scale. The scale, developed in 1932, allows respondents to specify their level of agreement to a statement.[46] The Likert scale dichotomizes a subject's opinion into an "agree" or "disagree" category. The 4-point Likert scale, which eliminates the middle category of the 5-point scale, will generally force a respondent to tip toward agreement or disagreement. Thus, we find the 4-point scale most useful for survey studies. Although the Likert scale is the most widely used scale in survey research, scientific investigators should be aware of the built-in biases of this scale. Respondents may attempt to avoid extreme responses (ie, strongly agree or strongly disagree), leading to central tendency bias. They may also attempt to portray themselves as agreeable, creating social desirability bias, or simply agree to the statement a[[parms resize(1),-pos(50,50),size(200,200),bgcol(156)]]se   biases, surveys will often word the same question in different ways to establish reproducibility of the results.

Although it may not appear to yield useful data, always allow "neither agree nor disagree," "don't know," "not-applicable," and "other" type of responses. These choices decrease frustration for those respondents who cannot choose a specific answer among the options given. They also allow the researcher to determine whether the person skipped the question or didn't answer

Example 1. Multiple choice (5-point Likert scale[46])
Which of the following best describes your overall hospital experience?
1. Very satisfactory
2. Satisfactory
3. Neither satisfactory nor unsatisfactory
4. Unsatisfactory
5. Very unsatisfactory

Example 2. Numeric open-ended
On a scale of 1-10, 1 being completely dissatisfied, and 10 being totally satisfied, how would you rate the customer service of our hospital? _____

Example 3. Text open-ended
What can our hospital do to improve patient care? _____

Example 4. Multiple choice (4-point Likert scale[46])
The customer service you encountered during the hospitalization was satisfactory.
1. Strongly agree
2. Agree
3. Disagree
4. Strongly disagree

Fig. 1. Common types of survey questions.

Table 2
Survey questions: key principles

Principle	Faulty Question	Revised Question
Example 1. Always check for bias in your questions.	Do you think this acne treatment: a) Improved your acne b) Had no effect c) Don't know	How would you describe your acne condition after treatment with this medication? a) Improved b) Had no effect c) Worse d) Not sure
Example 2. Avoid putting questions at the beginning of a survey if it can potentially bias the rest of the survey.	1. I view nurse practitioners as: 1. Competitors 2. Partners or colleagues 3. Subordinates 4. None of the above	Better placed at end of the survey
Example 3. Avoid asking two questions in one.	"Have you ever gone to a tanning salon or used a sunless tanning product?"	1. Have you ever used a sunless tanning product? a) Yes b) No 2. If you answered yes to #1, what brand(s) have you used? a) Brand X b) Brand Y c) Brand Z d) Don't remember
Example 4. Make sure all relevant alternatives are included in the list of response choices. Alphabetizing can be useful.	What brand of soap does your household most often use? 1. Dial 2. Oil of Olay 3. Dove 4. Ivory 5. Lever 2000 6. Irish Spring 7. Other (please list):	What brand of bar soap does your household most often use? 1. Dial 2. Dove 3. Irish Spring 4. Ivory 5. Lever 2000 6. Oil of Olay 7. Other (please list): 8. Don't use bar soap

Example 5. Avoid asking respondents to sort long lists; and do not use confusing tables that require subjects to add to 100 in their head.

Please rank the following 10 acne treatments based on how often you prescribe them: or Please estimate what % of your mild to moderate acne patients have been prescribed each of these 10 treatments in the last 12 months (Enter a number between 0 to 100 in each field, all answers should add to 100).

1. What are your top three prescribed medications for acne?
2. How often do you prescribe each: never, rarely, occasionally, frequently, very often?

Example 6. Avoid asking subjects to remember their previous answers.

If prior authorizations for topical retinoids were lifted, what would your new % of prescriptions be?

If prior authorizations for topical retinoids were lifted, how would it affect your frequency of prescriptions?
a) Increase prescribed retinoids
b) Not affect prescription patterns
c) Decrease prescribed retinoids

Example 7. Try to use word choices for respondents when addressing frequency of use. Presenting data that say 30% of people use acne pads 26%–50% of the time is cumbersome.

What percent of time do you incorporate a medicated/cleansing pad into your acne routine?
a) Never
b) 1%–25%
c) 26%–50%
d) 51%–75%
e) 76%–100%

How often do you use a medicated/cleansing pad in your daily acne routine?
a) Never
b) Rarely
c) Sometimes
d) Often
e) Always OR

How often do you use a medicated/cleansing pad in your daily acne routine?
a) Never (<1%)
b) Rarely (1%–33% of time)
c) Sometimes (24%–66% of time)
d) Often (67%–99% of time)
e) Always (100% of time)

Example 8. Avoid including answers that overlap.

In what type of setting do you practice?
a) Academic setting
b) Private setting
c) Hospital-affiliated

Which of the following best describes your practice:
a) Academic practice
b) Solo private dermatology practice
c) Group private dermatology practice
d) Group private multidisciplinary practice
e) Other, please specify

Example 9. Allow the use of n/a (not applicable) as an option, otherwise it can be unclear whether the subject skipped the question or if it was truly not applicable.

How effective do you find photodynamic therapy is for acne patients?
1. Very effective
2. Somewhat effective
3. Not effective

How effective do you find photodynamic therapy (PDT) is for acne patients?
1. Very effective
2. Somewhat effective
3. Not effective
4. Not sure
5. Don't use PDT

it, which in turn helps to establish the appropriate denominator for each question.

Investigators should also be aware of common errors to avoid when writing survey questions. These include using leading words in a question, asking two questions in one, not including all relevant alternatives as answer choices, and creating answers that are not mutually exclusive. **Table 2** shows examples of these common errors, the biases that occur, and how to rephrase these questions in a more effective manner.

General Tips for Limiting Error

To achieve the best possible outcome from a survey, investigators must make every attempt to limit error. In the previous sections, we touched on the importance of minimizing nonresponse error as well as error from bias. However, additional forms of error need to be addressed as well. Sampling error is the inherent error that results from measuring only a subset of the general population. Investigators can attain relatively low levels of sampling error by performing random surveys on large sample populations.[29,31] Coverage error results when members of a survey population are left out of the study. For example, if one wanted to generate a list of dermatologists practicing in a particular geographic area and used the phone book to sample, they might systematically miss dermatologists that practice at a large HMO and therefore are not listed in the phone book. Coverage error can be minimized with inclusive databases. However, given the rarity and difficulty of finding patients with certain dermatologic diseases, these forms of error can often be difficult to avoid. Finally, measurement error occurs when questions are not accurately or consistently interpreted by respondents. Limiting this form of error requires the development of clearly readable questions.[30]

GETTING PUBLISHED

Box 1 provides a general breakdown of the goals and requirements necessary for transferring survey research into publishable material. To begin, clearly documented institutional review board (IRB) or other appropriate human experimental ethics committee review should always have occurred prior to sending out a survey.[47] Additionally, a solid measurable hypothesis that addresses relevant, interesting issues for dermatologists is of the utmost importance. The hypothesis should be supported by the literature. Once the hypothesis has been formed, investigators need to build a survey with readable questions that will serve to directly address the hypothesis

---

Box 1
Guidelines for publication

1. Obtain and provide IRB approval
2. Find interesting, meaningful issues in dermatology to analyze
3. Develop a solid, measurable hypothesis
4. Support the hypothesis with literature
5. Produce readable, interpretable questions
6. Make survey available to publication
7. One survey should result in one publication
8. Address scope and degree of error in study

---

being proposed.[30,48] Furthermore, the survey should be made available in the publication for readers,[49] and one survey should generally translate into only one article. When publishing or presenting survey material, investigators must address the scope and degree of error in their report. These principles on publication should coincide with the guidelines outlined in the preceding sections (see **Box 1**).

The *Journal of the American Academy of Dermatology* (JAAD)[50] and *Archives of Dermatology*[51] both reference survey research in their authorship guidelines. *Archives of Dermatology* suggest only that a survey must have significant response rates.[51] The JAAD, however, provides specific authorship requirements. The journal necessitates IRB documentation, a copy of the survey instrument, approval for the use of lists used in the distribution of the survey, and an explanation for the survey's importance and validity.[50] These guidelines, while providing basic requirements for publication, will not suffice for achieving reviewer approval. As previously stressed, reviewers will look for a survey's accuracy and statistical significance as well as its contribution to the medical community.

PREVIOUS USE OF SURVEY RESEARCH IN DERMATOLOGY
Patient-Based Surveys

Surveys provide investigators with a powerful method for analyzing patient attitudes, preferences, and opinions. Without surveys, this information would otherwise be unavailable to the medical community. Skin diseases have the potential to have a significant impact on a patient's physical and psychologic well-being. Oftentimes, the patient's self-assessment of disease may not coincide with the physician's objective analysis. Numerous investigators have used the survey to answer questions regarding patient quality of life and satisfaction with treatments. Psoriasis,[1–3,6,7]

Table 3		
Survey research: topics covered in dermatologic publications		
Patient Based	**Physician Based**	**Residency, Fellowship, Community Based**
• Treatment satisfaction • Quality of life • Perception of symptoms • Patient self-reported risk factors • Comorbidities	• Medical knowledge • Patient management • Treatment preferences • Diagnosis patterns	• Training satisfaction • Evaluation process • Community opinions

atopic dermatitis,[13–15] bullous disease,[16,17] contact dermatitis,[18] acne,[52] vitiligo,[53] general chronic dermatologic disease,[54] and skin cancer[19,55] are just a few cutaneous diseases where surveys have been used to analyze patient opinions. Journals publish a wide variety of types of surveys (**Table 3**).

Physician-Based Surveys

Surveys have also been used to assess physician attitudes and beliefs on a wide variety of dermatologic topics. Investigators have used the instruments to analyze diagnostic patterns, treatment paradigms, and general knowledge for practicing dermatologists. The surveys have functioned to evaluate physician attitudes on psoriasis,[8,9] melanoma[20,21] and nonmelanoma skin cancer,[23,24] vaccinations,[56] and warts (see **Table 2**).[57] In this regard, the surveys have attempted to objectively analyze subjective opinions and practices of dermatologists (see **Table 3**).

Residency- and Fellowship-Based Surveys/ Community-based Surveys

Nondisease-related issues in dermatology have been evaluated with surveys as well. Issues such as teledermatology in residencies,[58] evaluation of dermatology fellowships,[25] teaching methods for dermoscopy,[26] and general satisfaction with residency training are just a few of the issues that have been analyzed.[27] Investigators have also surveyed the wider community or segments of the population (ie, teens) in relation to issues such as tanning and skin cancer.[28] The survey provides a solid option for measuring these subjective factors (see **Table 3**).

SUMMARY

Successfully published survey research has focused on a variety of topics in dermatology. Surveys can effectively provide necessary information on the opinions of patients, physicians, residents, and the general community, and ultimately impact clinical care. Many dermatologic journals have found survey research worth publication. This widely used research tool can provide important scientific information, particularly about attitudes and behaviors. Limiting error remains an essential issue to consider regardless of the survey type. Following the key guidelines outlined in this article will assist investigators in the optimal development and use of their surveys.

REFERENCES

1. Healy PJ, Helliwell PS. Psoriatic arthritis quality of life instrument: an assessment of sensitivity and response to change. J Rheumatol 2008;35(7):1359–61.
2. Gelfand JM, Kimball AB, Mostow EN, et al. Patient-reported outcomes and health-care resource utilization in patients with psoriasis treated with etanercept: continuous versus interrupted treatment. Value Health 2008;11(3):400–7.
3. Seikowski K, Gelbrich M, Harth W [Sexual self-reflection in patients with atopic dermatitis and psoriasis]. Hautarzt 2008;59(4):297–303 [in German].
4. Kilic A, Gulec MY, Gul U, et al. Temperament and character profile of patients with psoriasis. J Eur Acad Dermatol Venereol 2008;22(5):537–42.
5. Zamirska A, Reich A, Berny-Moreno J, et al. Vulvar pruritus and burning sensation in women with psoriasis. Acta Derm Venereol 2008;88(2):132–5.
6. Zachariae R, Zachariae CO, Lei U, et al. Affective and sensory dimensions of pruritus severity: associations with psychological symptoms and quality of life in psoriasis patients. Acta Derm Venereol 2008; 88(2):121–7.
7. Ciocon DH, Horn EJ, Kimball AB. Quality of life and treatment satisfaction among patients with psoriasis and psoriatic arthritis and patients with psoriasis only: results of the 2005 spring US National Psoriasis Foundation survey. Am J Clin Dermatol 2008;9(2):111–7.
8. Patel V, Horn EJ, Lobosco SJ, et al. Psoriasis treatment patterns: results of a cross-sectional survey of dermatologists. J Am Acad Dermatol 2008;58(6):964–9.
9. Augustin M, Kruger K, Radtke MA, et al. Disease severity, quality of life and health care in plaque-type psoriasis: a multicenter cross-sectional study in Germany. Dermatology 2008;216(4):366–72.

10. Weiss SC, Rehmus W, Kimball AB. An assessment of the cost-utility of therapy for psoriasis. Ther Clin Risk Manag 2006;2(3):325–8.

11. Hong J, Koo B, Koo J. The psychosocial and occupational impact of chronic skin disease. Dermatol Ther 2008;21(1):54–9.

12. Schmitt J, Csotonyi F, Bauer A, et al. Determinants of treatment goals and satisfaction of patients with atopic eczema. J Dtsch Dermatol Ges 2008;6(6):458–65.

13. Peroni DG, Piacentini GL, Bodini A, et al. Prevalence and risk factors for atopic dermatitis in preschool children. Br J Dermatol 2008;158(3):539–43.

14. Mozaffari H, Pourpak Z, Pourseyed S, et al. Quality of life in atopic dermatitis patients. J Microbiol Immunol Infect 2007;40(3):260–4.

15. Ganemo A, Svensson A, Lindberg M, et al. Quality of life in Swedish children with eczema. Acta Derm Venereol 2007;87(4):345–9.

16. Tabolli S, Mozzetta A, Antinone V, et al. The health impact of pemphigus vulgaris and pemphigus foliaceus assessed using the medical outcomes study 36-item short form health survey questionnaire. Br J Dermatol 2008;158(5):1029–34.

17. Gisondi P, Sampogna F, Annessi G, et al. Severe impairment of quality of life in Hailey-Hailey disease. Acta Derm Venereol 2005;85(2):132–5.

18. Rabin B, Fraidlin N. Patients with occupational contact dermatitis in Israel: quality of life and social implications. Soc Work Health Care 2007;45(2):97–111.

19. Chren MM, Sahay AP, Bertenthal DS, et al. Quality-of-life outcomes of treatments for cutaneous basal cell carcinoma and squamous cell carcinoma. J Invest Dermatol 2007;127(6):1351–7.

20. Grange F, Vitry F, Granel-Brocard F, et al. Variations in management of stage I to stage III cutaneous melanoma: a population-based study of clinical practices in France. Arch Dermatol 2008;144(5):629–36.

21. Saez-de-Ocariz M, Sosa-de-Martinez C, Duran-McKinster C, et al. Cutaneous melanoma in private vs. public practices of Mexican dermatologists. Int J Dermatol 2008;47(6):637–9.

22. Cashin RP, Lui P, Machado M, et al. Advanced cutaneous malignant melanoma: a systematic review of economic and quality-of-life studies. Value Health 2008;11(2):259–71.

23. John Chen G, Yelverton CB, Polisetty SS, et al. Treatment patterns and cost of nonmelanoma skin cancer management. Dermatol Surg 2006;32(10):1266–71.

24. Gudi V, Ormerod AD, Dawn G, et al. Management of basal cell carcinoma by surveyed dermatologists in Scotland. Clin Exp Dermatol 2006;31(5):648–52.

25. Freeman SR, Nelson C, Lundahl K, et al. Similar deficiencies in procedural dermatology and dermatopathology fellow evaluation despite different periods of ACGME accreditation: results of a national survey. Dermatol Surg 2008;34(7):873–6 [discussion 76–7].

26. Argenziano G, Zalaudek I, Soyer HP. Which is the most reliable method for teaching dermoscopy for melanoma diagnosis to residents in dermatology? Br J Dermatol 2004;151(2):512–3.

27. Webb JM, Rye B, Fox L, et al. State of dermatology training: the residents' perspective. J Am Acad Dermatol 1996;34(6):1067–71.

28. Lazovich D, Stryker JE, Mayer JA, et al. Measuring nonsolar tanning behavior: indoor and sunless tanning. Arch Dermatol 2008;144(2):225–30.

29. Groves RM. Survey errors and survey costs. New York: Wiley; 1989.

30. Dillman DA. Mail and Internet surveys: the tailored design method. 2nd edition. New York: John Wiley & Sons, Inc.; 2007.

31. Salant P, Dillman DA. How to conduct your own survey. New York: Wiley; 1994.

32. Blau PM. Exchange and power in social life. New York: Wiley; 1964.

33. James JM, Bolstein R. Large monetary incentives and their effect on mail survey response rates. Public Opin Q 1992;56:442–3.

34. de Leeuw ED, Hox JJ, Kef S, et al. The effects of response-stimulating factors on response rates and data quality in mail surveys: a test of Dillman's total design methods. J Off Stat 1988;4:241–9.

35. Asch DA, Jedrziewski MK, Christakis NA. Response rates to mail surveys published in medical journals. J Clin Epidemiol 1997;50(10):1129–36.

36. Scott C. Research on mail surveys. J R Stat Soc 1961;124:143–205.

37. Heberlein TA, Baumgartner R. Factors affecting response rates to mailed questionnaires: a quantitative analysis of the published literature. Am Sociol Rev 1978;43:447–62.

38. Edwards P, Roberts I, Clarke M, et al. Increasing response rates to postal questionnaires: systematic review. BMJ 2002;324(7347):1183–5.

39. Edwards P, Cooper R, Roberts I, et al. Meta-analysis of randomised trials of monetary incentives and response to mailed questionnaires. J Epidemiol Community Health 2005;59(11):987–99.

40. Halpern SD, Ubel PA, Berlin JA, et al. Randomized trial of 5 dollars versus 10 dollars monetary incentives, envelope size, and candy to increase physician response rates to mailed questionnaires. Med Care 2002;40(9):834–9.

41. Asch DA, Christakis NA. Different response rates in a trial of two envelop styles in mail survey research. Epidemiology 1994;5(3):364–5.

42. Sharp L, Cochran C, Cotton SC, et al. Enclosing a pen with a postal questionnaire can significantly increase the response rate. J Clin Epidemiol 2006;59(7):747–54.

43. Dillman DA. Mail and telephone surveys: the tailored design method. New York: Wiley; 1978.

44. Leece P, Bhandari M, Sprague S, et al. Internet versus mailed questionnaires: a controlled comparison (2). J Med Internet Res 2004;6(4):e39.

45. Akl EA, Maroun N, Klocke RA, et al. Electronic mail was not better than postal mail for surveying residents and Faculty. J Clin Epidemiol 2005;58(4):425–9.

46. Likert R. A technique for the measurement of attitudes. Arch Psychol 1932;140:5–55.

47. Orvis AK, Dellavalle RP. Institutional review board approval for surveys: why it is necessary. J Am Acad Dermatol 2008;59(4):718–9.

48. Payne SL. The art of asking questions. Princeton (NJ): Princeton University Press.; 1951.

49. Schilling LM, Kozak K, Lundahl K, et al. Inaccessible novel questionnaires in published medical research: hidden methods, hidden costs. Am J Epidemiol 2006;164(12):1141–4.

50. Journal of the American Academy of Dermatology Web site. Information for authors. Available at: http://www.journals.elsevierhealth.com/periodicals/ymjd/authorinfo. Accessed January 8, 2009.

51. Archives of Dermatology Web site. Information for authors. Available at: http://archderm.ama-assn.org/misc/ifora.dtl. Accessed January 8, 2009.

52. Augustin M, Reich C, Schaefer I, et al. Development and validation of a new instrument for the assessment of patient-defined benefit in the treatment of acne. J Dtsch Dermatol Ges 2008;6(2):113–20.

53. Sukan M, Maner F. The problems in sexual functions of vitiligo and chronic urticaria patients. J Sex Marital Ther 2007;33(1):55–64.

54. Evers AW, Duller P, van de Kerkhof PC, et al. The impact of chronic skin disease on daily life (ISDL): a generic and dermatology-specific health instrument. Br J Dermatol 2008;158(1):101–8.

55. Blanchard CM, Courneya KS, Stein K. Cancer survivors' adherence to lifestyle behavior recommendations and associations with health-related quality of life: results from the American Cancer Society's SCS-II. J Clin Oncol 2008;26(13):2198–204.

56. Dellavalle RP, Heilig LF, Francis SO, et al. What dermatologists do not know about smallpox vaccination: results from a worldwide electronic survey. J Invest Dermatol 2006;126(5):986–9.

57. Henderson Z, Irwin KL, Montano DE, et al. Anogenital warts knowledge and counseling practices of us clinicians: results from a national survey. Sex Transm Dis 2007;34(9):644–52.

58. Scheinfeld N, Fisher M, Genis P, et al. Evaluating patient acceptance of a teledermatology link of an urban urgent-care dermatology clinic run by residents with board certified dermatologists. Skinmed 2003;2(3):159–62.

Social Internet Sites as a Source of Public Health Information

Karl Vance, BS[a], William Howe, MD[a],
Robert P. Dellavalle, MD, PhD, MSPH[a,b,c],*

KEYWORDS

- Viral marketing • Web 2.0 • YouTube • Twitter
- MySpace • Facebook • Social media

Patients rely on the Internet more frequently than their physicians as a source of health care information, and emerging social media Web sites play an increasing role in online health searches.[1] Socially oriented sites, such as YouTube, Facebook, MySpace, Twitter, and Second Life®, comprise part of the user-generated content constituting Web 2.0 and are popular particularly among Americans aged 18 to 30, two thirds of whom say they visit the sites frequently.[2–4] A health-specific social Web site, http://www.patientslikeme.com, even allows patients who have similar illnesses to communicate and share medical experiences.[5]

SOCIAL MEDIA MARKETING

"Social media marketing" encompasses advertising and promotional efforts that use social media Web sites.[6] It is a form of viral marketing, a term coined by Harvard professor Jeffrey F. Rayport in 1996, to illustrate how a message spreads through an online community rapidly and effortlessly.[7] The content of social media marketing campaigns often is user generated; companies, such as General Motors, JetBlue, and Sony, have sponsored contests for viewers to submit videos promoting their products, simultaneously involving customers in the marketing process and obtaining creative new ideas virtually free of charge. Creative videos often are then widely disseminated by viewers via e-mail and hyperlinks on personal Web sites. Analogously, in the dermatology community, the Sulzberger Institute for Dermatologic Education[8] is sponsoring an Internet contest for the best video promoting sun safe behavior.

SOCIAL NETWORKING WEB SITES

In contrast to the music and film industries, which rapidly adapted social media marketing, this medium remains underused by public health professionals despite its low cost and wide reach. MySpace and Facebook pages for musical bands and new movies abound, encouraging fans to listen to new tracks or view theatrical trailers. Political campaigns also reach out to young adults through social networking sites: 8% of people polled under age 30 became an online "friend" of one of the presidential candidates in the 2008 election.[4] Physicians similarly could be "friended." The young adult demographic using social media sites are attractive to media for spreading public health messages targeting this population, such as sun safety awareness, tobacco cessation, and human papillomavirus vaccination education. Just as young adults can "friend" their favorite

Supported by University of Colorado Denver, School of Medicine, Colorado Health Informatics Collaboration interdisciplinary academic enrichment funds (RPD) and by National Cancer Institute grant K-07 CA92550 (RPD).

a Department of Dermatology, University of Colorado at Denver and Health Sciences Center, P.O. Box 6510, Mail Stop F703, Aurora, CO 80045, USA
b Department of Veterans Affairs Medical Center, 1055 Clermont Street, #165, Denver, CO, USA
c Colorado School of Public Health, 13001 E. 17th Place, Campus Box B119, Aurora, CO, 80045, USA
* Corresponding author. Colorado School of Public Health, 13001 E. 17th Place, Campus Box B119, Aurora, CO 80045.
E-mail address: robert.dellavalle@ucdenver.edu (R.P. Dellavalle).

Dermatol Clin 27 (2009) 133–136
doi:10.1016/j.det.2008.11.010

band, movie, or political candidate, they could add a link on their personal page to a skin health site with updates on acne treatment and other health messages.

YOUTUBE

More than 100 million videos are viewed on YouTube daily, and that number continues to rise.[9] Several recent public health studies have looked at the content of videos hosted on YouTube that have tobacco and human papillomavirus vaccination messages.[10–12] Researchers point out the potential power YouTube holds for personal health decision making. A cursory search on YouTube for the term "Accutane" results in 87 hits with titles ranging from "An Accutane Story: The Chapstick Chronicles" to "Accutane is POISON! DO NOT USE IT!!!!" The majority of videos are mainly positive accounts by Accutane users sharing their personal experiences with other viewers. An overview of the top three videos by relevance is provided in **Table 1**.

A similar YouTube search for the term "Botox" returns 2750 videos; the top three videos sorted by relevance are provided in **Table 1**. Many of the top Botox videos actually are advertisements posted by Botox providers. These promotional videos often include footage of Botox injections and personal testimonials by patients receiving treatments. Frequently, the patients receive discounts for their participation, raising ethical

Table 1
A summary of the top three videos ranked by relevance[a] resulting from a YouTube search for "Accutane" or "Botox" on August 15, 2008

Video Title	No. of Views	Time Since Posted	No. of Comments	Description
"Accutane" results				
"My Acne Story (Accutane)"	16,264	10 months	249	An Accutane patient's personal story of how the medication helped him, a warning of side effects, and a request for other patients to share their experiences.
"Accutane Before and After"	11,939	4 months	69	An Accutane patient's before and after photos.
"Accutane"	17,188	2 years	187	An advertisement for Accutane suggesting that Accutane will help you get out and participate in life.
"Botox" results				
"Learn about Botox injection- Upper face The Institute"	79,700	21 months	70	Video of botox injections followed by a smiling patient, phone number, and Web site address of the provider's office.
"Alexis gets quarterly dose of botox" (video contains adult language)	24,325	15 months	32	Video of a patient joking before and during a Botox procedure, mentioning the provider's name.
"Kelly Ripa—to botox or to not Botox?"	29,976	16 months	11	Morning talk show host Kelly Ripa talks about a book describing alternatives to Botox and states that she has not had any injections.

[a] Relevance refers to the default ranking for YouTube queries and is determined by a proprietary algorithm.

questions.[13] Paid testimonials may not reflect patient experience accurately. Social media marketing currently lies outside the realm of governmental regulation. It is important for the dermatology community to be aware of dermatologists advertising on these new media. Such monitoring will promote the integrity of the profession.

SECOND LIFE®

Second Life® is an incarnation of Web 2.0 that creates a virtual realm in which people can interact through 3-D characters, named "avatars."[14] The site serves as a physician teaching tool for trainees and patients and a new forum for exchanging scientific information and holding scientific meetings. Second Life allows users to interact in many formats, including audio, video, images, and text, and brings people "together" in virtual space while they remain geographically distant.[15] A dermatology Second Life® realm could offer patients a site with expert opinions from across the globe or an online support group for specific diseases.

TWITTER

Microblogging is another expanding feature of Web 2.0 that enables users to rapidly provide others with video, image, and text updates. Twitter[16] is the most prominent site, with more than 3,300,000 registered users,[17] although other microblogging sites exist, such as http://jaiku. com,[18] and MySpace and Facebook offer similar features in the form of "updates." Companies, such as JetBlue, Whole Foods Market, and H&R Block, are using Twitter to reach their customers with new offers and to answer questions and concerns.[19] Microblogging also has potential as a medical support group format; currently a Twitter site exists for mothers of children who have attention deficit disorder.[20] Physicians could reach their patients through Twitter to update them with therapeutic advancements, to answer disease-related questions, or simply to remind a large group of engaged consumers to wear their daily sunscreen.

CHALLENGES

Social media marketing has its own set of regulatory challenges.[21–23] Authorship is difficult to determine, sources rarely are provided, and users may post their personal opinions as comments. The Health On the Net (HON) Foundation has created a set of eight major criteria, such as stated authorship, patient privacy, and attribution of information, that Web sites must meet to display the "HONcode" logo.[24] Criteria such as these cannot be applied, however, to social media Web sites, and thoughtful action should be taken to provide patients with sound medical advice within online social networks.

REFERENCES

1. Sarasohn-Kahn J. The wisdom of patients: health care meets online social media. Available at: http://www. chcf.org/topics/chronicdisease/index.cfm?itemID= 133631. Accessed January 5, 2009.
2. Alexa. United States Alexa top 500 sites. Available at: http://www.alexa.com/site/ds/top_sites?cc=US&ts_ mode=country&lang=none. Accessed January 5, 2009.
3. Johnson K, Freeman S, Dellavalle RP. Wikis: the application of Web 2.0. Arch Dermatol 2007; 143(8):1065–6.
4. The Pew Research Center for The People & The Press Internet's broader role in campaign 2008: social networking and online videos take off. Available at: http://www.people-press.org/report/384/internets-broader-role-in-campaign-2008. Accessed January 5, 2009.
5. Patientslikeme.com. Available at: http://www. patientslikeme.com/. Accessed January 5, 2009.
6. Bosman J. Chevy tries a write-your-own-ad approach, and the potshots fly. NY Times April 4, 2006. Available at: http://www.nytimes.com/2006/ 04/04/business/media/04adco.html?_r=1&;oref=slogin. Accessed January 5, 2009.
7. Rayport J. The Virus of Marketing. Fast Company 1996:6. Available at: http://www.fastcompany.com/ magazine/06/virus.html. www.fastcompany.com/mag azine/06/virus.html. Accessed January 5, 2009.
8. American Academy of Dermatology. The Sulzberger Institute. Available at: http://www.aad.org/education/ grants/sulzberger_inst.htm. Accessed January 5, 2009.
9. Hof R. YouTube: 100 million videos a day. Business Week. July 14, 2006. Available at: http://www.busi nessweek.com/the_thread/techbeat/archives/2006/ 07/youtube_100_mil.html. Accessed January 5, 2009.
10. Ache K, Wallace L. Human papillomavirus vaccination coverage on YouTube. Am J Prev Med 2008. Pre-publication copy downloaded August 9, 2008.
11. Keelan J, Pavri-Garcia V, Tomlinson G, et al. YouTube as a source of information on immunization: a content analysis. JAMA 2007;21:2482–4.
12. Freeman B, Chapman S. Is YouTube telling or selling you something? Tobacco content on the video-sharing website YouTube. Tob Control 2007;16:207–10.
13. Ellin A. Coming Soon to YouTube: My-Facelift. Available at: http://www.nytimes.com/2008/06/26/fashion/ 26SKIN.html. Accessed on January 5, 2009.

14. Second Life. Available at: http://www.secondlife. com. Accessed January 5, 2009.

15. Huang S, Boulos M, Dellavalle R. Will your next poster session be in second life? EMBO Rep 2008; 9(6):496–9.

16. Twitter. What is Twitter? Available at: http://www.twit ter.com. Accessed January 5, 2009.

17. Twitter directory. Available at: http://www.twitdir.com. Accessed January 5, 2009.

18. Jaiku. Welcome to Jaiku. Available at: http://www. jaiku.com. Accessed January 5, 2009.

19. Mardesich J. Business uses for twitter. Available at: http://technology.inc.com/networking/articles/ 200809/twitter.html. Accessed January 5, 2009.

20. ADDmoms on twitter. Available at: http://www.twitter. com/ADDmoms. Accessed January 5, 2009.

21. Greenberg L, D'Andrea G, Lorence D. Setting the public agenda for online health search: a white paper and action agenda. J Med Internet Res 2004;6(2):e18. Available at: http://www.jmir.org/ 2004/2/e18. Accessed January 5, 2009.

22. Connecting with patients, overcoming uncertainty. White paper by TNS media intelligence/cymfony, envision solutions, LLC, and seyfarth shaw LLP; September 2007. Available at: http://www.seyfarth. com/dir_docs/news_item/1d21aaf1-4ad5-4e22- af28-af3feea533e6_documentupload.pdf. Accessed August 9, 2008.

23. Silberg W, Lundberg G, Musacchio R. Assessing, controlling, and assuring the quality of medical information on the internet. JAMA 1997;277: 1244–5.

24. HON code of conduct (HONcode) for medical and health web sites. Available at: http://www.hon.ch/ HONcode/Conduct.html. Accessed January 5, 2009.

Comorbidities in Dermatology

Marlies Wakkee, MD, Tamar Nijsten, MD, PhD*

KEYWORDS

- Comorbidities • Epidemiology • Psoriasis
- Atopic dermatitis • Vitiligo • Non-melanoma skin cancer

There is no universally accepted definition for the term comorbidity. Traditionally, comorbidity has been defined as a medical condition coexisting with the primary disease either as a current or past condition.[1] Wikipedia defines comorbidity as the "the effect of all other diseases an individual patient might have other than the primary disease of interest."[2] Comorbidities should be distinguished from diseases with a common immunologic pathogenesis (eg, mixed connective tissue diseases and related skin conditions) or dermatoses strongly associated with specific (internal) diseases (eg, erythema nodosum and sarcoidosis or inflammatory bowel disease).

The association between dermatologic diseases and comorbidities is often complex and multifactorial making it difficult to demonstrate direct relationships (**Fig. 1**). Life style factors, impaired health-related quality of life, depression, therapeutic interventions, and varying use of medical care may confound an association between a skin disease and comorbidity. Also, several biases, such as detection bias (ie, patients with a skin disease are more likely to be diagnosed with another disease while visiting their physician for their dermatosis) may affect observational studies results.

The presence of comorbidities in dermatology is of interest for various reasons. From a preventative perspective, a skin disease can be an early marker of systemic disease, and therefore, identify patients who are at risk of having other, more life-threatening diseases. An association between a skin disease and comorbidities may influence clinical management (eg, multidisciplinary approach and

treatment options). Ideally, treatments are selected that improve both conditions simultaneously. However, comorbidities may also be a contra-indication for therapies indicated for the skin disease or drugs used in the treatment of the comorbidity may interact with the dermatologic therapy.

Comorbidities impact health-related quality of life (HRQOL) in patients with a dermatologic condition.[3] Knowledge about the association between a dermatosis and another disease may increase the understanding of the shared pathogenesis of both diseases.

The objective of this review is to provide an overview of comorbidities in dermatology. The focus will be on direct and indirect (eg, therapy or life-style related) associations, the likelihood of the association, and possible consequences in daily practice.

PSORIASIS

Most research on comorbidities in dermatology has been conducted among patients with psoriasis.[4] Psoriatic arthritis, cardiovascular diseases or the metabolic syndrome, malignancies, infections, auto-immune diseases, and depression are all associated with psoriasis.

Psoriatic Arthritis

A well-known comorbidity in psoriasis is psoriatic arthritis (PsA). The prevalence among patients with psoriasis varies from 6% to 40%, depending on the population studied, but is likely to be about 10%.[5] PsA is a seronegative spondylarthropathy and there are five subtypes: arthritis of the distal

Department of Dermatology, Erasmus Medical Centre, P.O. Box 2040, 3000 CA Rotterdam, The Netherlands
* Corresponding author.
E-mail address: t.nijsten@erasmusmc.nl (T. Nijsten).

Dermatol Clin 27 (2009) 137–147
doi:10.1016/j.det.2008.11.013

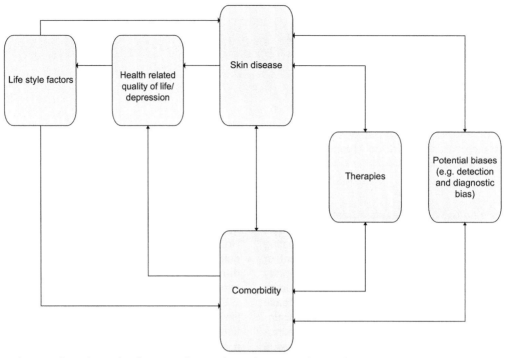

Fig. 1. The complex relationship between dermatologic diseases and comorbidities.

interphalangeal joints, asymmetric oligoarthritis, symmetric polyarthritis, spondylitis, and arthritis mutilans.[6] The joint complaints generally occur 7- to 10- years after the onset of psoriasis, but may also present themselves without cutaneous signs of psoriasis in about 10% of the cases. Patients with early onset psoriasis, severe disease, nail changes, and pustular types of psoriasis have the highest likelihood of developing PsA. No serologic marker exists for PsA. The simplest and frequently used diagnostic criteria for PsA includes the presence of inflammatory arthritis, psoriasis, and the absence of serologic tests for rheumatoid factor.[6] More recently, the more specific Classification criteria for Psoriatic Arthritis (CASPAR) have been introduced, which also included features such as family history of psoriasis, nail dystrophy, and juxta-articular new bone formation.[7] Most importantly, PsA is diagnosed by excluding other forms of seronegative arthritis (ie, absence of serum markers such as rheumatoid factor).[8] PsA can result in extensive irreversible joint damage[9] that may be prevented by early detection and treatment.[10,11]

Cardiovascular Disease

Psoriasis is a chronic inflammatory skin disorder in which many different inflammatory cells are involved. T-lymphocytes play a major role in this network, predominantly releasing type 1 cytokines, such as interferon-gamma, tumor necrosis factor-alpha, and interleukin-2, at the site of inflammation.[12] These cytokines further stimulate T-lymphocyte proliferation, the production of cytokines by T-lymphocytes and macrophages, chemokine release from macrophages, and the expression of adhesion molecules on vascular endothelial cells. The inflammation leads to oxidative stress that may result in systemic consequences.[13] High levels of oxidants stimulate the formation of atherosclerotic lesions in the vessel walls that may lead to a higher cardiovascular disease risk.

Cardiovascular diseases and the metabolic syndrome, which comprises the presence of three, or more, of five cardiovascular risk factors, such as obesity, increased cholesterol and triglycerides, hypertension, and glucose intolerance, have recently recaptured the attention in psoriasis research. As early as 1973, an increased prevalence of occlusive vascular disease among psoriasis inpatients compared with other dermatologic inpatients (11.5% versus 5.0%) was reported.[14] In 1986, a Swedish cross-sectional study suggested an association between psoriasis and hypertension, but this was not confirmed in a large, United States, prospective cohort study.[15,16] Another Swedish study demonstrated a 50% greater risk of death from cardiovascular disease, among patients who were treated at least once as a psoriasis inpatient, compared with the general population.[17] In contrast, the overall risk for cardiovascular death was slightly decreased among outpatients with psoriasis (standardized mortality ratio = 0.94; 95% Confidence Interval [CI] 0.89-0.99). The findings that hospitalized patients with psoriasis, especially those severely affected, are at increased risk, were confirmed in a German retrospective- cohort study of 581 cases and an Italian case control study including 338 patients.[18,19] Two prospective, population-based cohort studies from the United Kingdom and the United States demonstrated that patients with psoriasis have higher risks of myocardial infarction, angina, atherosclerosis, peripheral vascular diseases, and stroke.[20,21] The relative risk for myocardial infarction was greatest among young patients with severe psoriasis; a 30-year-old patient with severe psoriasis had an adjusted relative risk of 3.10 (95% CI 1.98-4.86) for myocardial infarction compared with the general population. From this same UK General Practice Research Database (GPRD), a study showed a strong association between severe psoriasis and cardiovascular risk factors like diabetes, hypertension, hyperlipidemia, obesity, and smoking.[22] After adjusting for the available information on traditional cardiovascular risk factors, these associations persisted in case of diabetes (Odds Ratio [OR] =1.62; 95% CI 1.30-2.01), smoking (OR 1.31; 95% CI 1.17-1.47), and an increased body mass index (OR for BMI>30 = 1.79; 95% CI 1.55-2.05). In a large prospective cohort study of almost 80,000 United States nurses, increased measures of adiposity (waist circumference, hip circumference, and waist- to-hip ratio), and weight gain were strong risk factors for incident psoriasis, suggesting that weight gain precedes the development of psoriasis, which is consistent with the findings of an Italian case control study.[23,24]

Two recent population based database studies that included pharmacy data did not confirm the association between psoriasis and treatment of cardiovascular disease. In a study using the data from the UK GPRD, patients with psoriasis were not more exposed to antihypertensive drugs before diagnosis of psoriasis.[25] In a Dutch population-based study using a pharmacy database, the 5-year prevalence exposure of cardiovascular and antidiabetic drugs were compared between patients with psoriasis and controls.[26] This study showed that patients with psoriasis were significantly more likely to have used antihypertensives, anticoagulant and antiplatelet agents, digoxin, nitrates, lipid lowering and antidiabetic drugs.

However, after adjusting for the number of unique drugs used in the history, which were used as a proxy for the consumption of health care, psoriasis was no longer associated with any of these drug classes suggesting that medical surveillance bias may have affected the study findings.

In summary, most but not all epidemiologic studies suggest that patients with psoriasis are at increased risk of cardiovascular disease. The absolute risk increase seems to be modest (about 20% to 30%) compared with the baseline risk in the general population. However, it remains challenging to differentiate whether the risk is due to the chronic inflammatory status of patients with psoriasis or other factors, such as different lifestyles, impaired HRQOL, prior drug exposures, and increased medical surveillance (**Fig. 1**). Prospective observational studies, including patients with incident psoriasis and all possible confounders, or randomized clinical studies are warranted to further explore the important association between psoriasis and cardiovascular disease.

The clinical implications for the current care of patients with psoriasis have been discussed among a group of experts in the United States.[27] Their advice was to follow the recommendations of the American Heart Association to screen for risk factors from as early as age 20, to repeat this at least once every 2 years from age 40, and to advise lifestyle modifications as first-line therapy when appropriate.

Malignancies

Several epidemiologic studies have suggested that patients with psoriasis are significantly more likely to develop nonmelanoma skin cancer (NMSC), lymphoma, and cancer of the lung, larynx, pharynx, liver, pancreas, female breast, vulva, penis, bladder and kidney.[28–30] Although chronic inflammation of the skin may decrease the risk of skin cancer because of increased cutaneous immunosurveillance, the incidence of squamous cell carcinoma (SCC), and to a lesser extent basal cell carcinoma (BCC), is increased in patients with psoriasis. This increased risk of NMSC seems primarily related to carcinogenic treatment exposures, such as high-dose psoralen plus ultraviolet A (PUVA), and to a lesser extent, of UVB.[31] The antipsoriatic therapy cyclosporine, especially after PUVA exposure, increases the risk of NMSC. The PUVA follow-up study showed an increased risk of melanoma in patients treated with PUVA, which is greater in patients exposed to high doses of PUVA and increases with the passage of time.[32] The carcinogenicity of coal tar has been shown in animal studies and in occupational settings.[33] Whether dermatologic use of coal tar as a monotherapy actually increases the risk of skin tumors and other malignancies is unknown.

In addition to agents used for psoriasis treatment, psoriasis has been associated with life-style factors, such as increased alcohol consumption and smoking, that are risk factors for oral cavity, esophagus, liver, pancreas, lung, kidney and breast cancer.[34] Two large cohort studies that followed up inpatients with psoriasis confirmed smoking and alcohol-related causes of death led to excess mortality.[28,35]

Several studies suggest an association between psoriasis and lymphoma with increasing risks for those severely affected by psoriasis.[28,36,37] A population-based study using the UK GPRD demonstrated an increased risk of about a third of developing any kind of lymphoma. The highest relative risks were observed for cutaneous T-cell lymphoma (adjusted relative risk=4.34 [95% CI 2.89-6.52]).[36,37] Caution is needed in the interpretation of these findings because the exposure to psoriasis therapies that may increase the risk of lymphoma (eg, cyclosporine and methotrexate) were not assessed and the results may have been affected by a misclassification bias (ie, patients having cutaneous T-cell lymphoma may have initially been misdiagnosed with psoriasis resulting in false positive psoriasis cases with a lymphoma). In a prospective cohort of 1380 patients treated with PUVA, only those with 36 months or more exposure of methotrexate developed significantly more lymphomas than expected (incidence rate ratio, 4.39; 95% CI, 1.59-12.06).[38] The possible effect of psoriasis therapies on the development of hematological malignancies is also suggested by a postmarketing study of cyclosporine.[39] Although the available studies suggest patients with psoriasis are at an increased risk of hematological malignancies, this association might be explained by an increased baseline risk, prior drug use, or misclassification. Further documentation about the baseline risk of lymphomas in patients with psoriasis would be valuable because biological therapies might increase lymphoma risk in this population.[40]

Infections

Several micro-organisms have been associated with provoking or exacerbating psoriasis. The strongest evidence exists for the induction of guttate psoriasis by a tonsillar Streptococcus pyogenes infection. The first case report of this association was published more than a century ago and more than 50 years ago, a study reported that in two thirds of patients with guttate psoriasis, there is a history of an acute sore throat 1- to 2-weeks before the eruption and serologic evidence of a recent streptococcal infection.[41] This observation has been confirmed by several other studies and some indicate that streptococcal throat infections can also cause exacerbation of chronic plaque psoriasis.[42]

An Austrian study showed that patients colonized with the toxin-positive S. aureus had a significantly higher psoriasis area and severity index score than patients with toxin negative S. aureus or without bacterial colonization.[43] In practice, secondary infections of chronic psoriasis plaques are rarely seen. This was confirmed by a large epidemiologic study on disease concomitance in psoriasis, which revealed that patients with psoriasis have an increased resistance to bacterial and viral infections compared with controls and patients with atopic dermatitis.[44] Approximately 30% of patients with atopic dermatitis suffered from either bacterial or viral infections, while this complication occurred in 7% of patients with psoriasis. These results may be related to the increased expression of antimicrobial peptides and proteins (AMPs) in psoriatic skin.[45,46] AMPs are involved in the innate defense against bacterial infections and clinical expression of these natural antibiotics correlate with the susceptibility to skin infections.

Psoriasis is associated with an increased beta-defensin genomic copy number.[47] Beta-defensins have broad-spectrum antimicrobial activities and proinflammatory properties. The variation in gene dosage may affect the development of infections and inflammatory diseases, which can contribute to the psoriasis susceptibility and the low prevalence of skin infections.

In contrast to cutaneous infections, systemic infections in patients with psoriasis are not well documented. A large Swedish population-based cohort study, which followed patients for a decade, found significantly more hospitalizations for pneumonia and systemic viral infections among patients with psoriasis compared with the general population, without taking systemic therapy exposure into consideration.[15] A few small retrospective case series that assessed postoperative infections after orthopedic surgery in patients with psoriasis have shown inconsistent findings: a case control study showed that 18% (15/85) of patients with postoperative infections had psoriasis and only 1% (2/202) of those without infections and concluded that psoriasis is a risk factor for postoperative infections after hip replacement surgery, but not for knee prosthesis.[48] Otherwise, severe immunodeficiency in human immunodeficiency virus

(HIV) may also trigger or exacerbate psoriasis.[49] The manifestations of psoriasis in patients with HIV vary. Usually it presents itself as the first clinical manifestation of HIV, although it can also appear in the advanced stages of HIV when it has progressed to AIDS.[50] The pathogenesis of psoriasis in HIV disease is not fully understood, but among Chinese patients with HIV, a significant association was found with the HLA-Cw*0602 allele.[51] Immune reconstitution by effective antiretroviral therapy has shown to significantly improve psoriasis.[52]

Immunosuppressive or immunomodulatory antipsoriatic therapies also increase the risk of systemic infections in patients with psoriasis. Methotrexate has been reported to cause reactivation of latent tuberculosis (TB) infection when used for the treatment of psoriasis. For cyclosporine, the development of TB has only been described in patients with transplants exposed to high doses of this drug.[53,54] Since the introduction of anti-TNF antibody therapies, several studies showed an increased risk of severe infections in these patients, of which tuberculosis is one of the most important.[40,55] Excluding latent TB and follow up of infectious signs is important in patients on immunosuppressive drugs, including the biologics. Evidence-based medicine on the role of vaccinations in patients with psoriasis using immunosupressants is still limited. A recent consensus statement, based on the available literature and expert opinions, advices standard vaccination before therapy initiation and annual inactivated influenza vaccine for patients on biologic agents until more long-term, follow-up evidence is available.[56] Live or live-attenuated vaccines should be avoided once one of these therapies has been initiated.

Others

A case-control study among 136 patients with inflammatory bowel diseases showed that psoriasis was more common among relatives of patients than in the controls (9.6% versus. 2.2%), which may be due to the genetic linkage with HLA B27 of these disorders.[57] The association between asymptomatic celiac disease and psoriasis remains controversial, which may be because of the high prevalence of antigliadin antibodies in the general population, or low specificity of these antibodies compared with those directed against transglutaminase.[58–60] A case-control study that included more than 12,500 patients with psoriasis, suggested that after adjusting for potential confounders, patients with psoriasis were about 25% more likely to develop chronic obstructive pulmonary disease than their matched controls.[61] Other diseases, such as gout or fatty liver disease, may primarily be caused by altered lifestyle factors.

ATOPIC DERMATITIS
Asthma and Allergic Rhinitis

The clinical signs of atopic dermatitis are frequently a harbinger of a well-described sequence of other atopic disorders, such as asthma and allergic rhinitis, the so-called "atopic march." These associations were confirmed in several large, well-designed longitudinal, observational studies, which provided evidence that approximately half of the patients with atopic dermatitis will develop asthma and two thirds will develop allergic rhinitis.[62] Severe atopic dermatitis and elevated serum IgE levels were found to be among the strongest risk factors for subsequent development of these allergic comorbidities.[63,64] Atopic diseases are also characterized by elevated IgE, peripheral and lesional eosinophilia, type 2 cytokines, epithelial dysfunction, similar allergenic triggers, and affected chromosomal regions.[65] The proposed mechanism that appears to induce the "atopic march" is epicutaneous sensitization through the barrier of disrupted skin, which induces a T helper 2 response in the skin.[66] The memory T helper 2 cells then migrate through the circulatory system to various sites, including the nasal and lung mucosa, promoting an allergic response in the airways after subsequent inhalation of these allergens.

There are studies suggesting that early intervention in atopic dermatitis with oral antihistamines might slow down the progression to allergic rhinitis and asthma.[67,68] Data on whether early anti-inflammatory treatment prevents the onset of asthma or merely delays its onset are not available.

Infections

Skin in patients with atopic dermatitis is frequently affected by bacterial colonization and recurrent skin infections by bacterial, fungal, and viral pathogens. The high rate of S. aureus infections is related to the increased ability of this bacteria to adhere to the skin of patients with atopic dermatitis, which may be explained by skin barrier dysfunction, an increased synthesis of the extracellular matrix adhesins for S. aureus, and a deficiency in the production of endogenous antimicrobial peptides.[69,70] In vitro studies observed that both extrinsic factors, such as cytokines and cell-autonomous differences, can influence the level of expression of genes involved in cutaneous inflammation and host defense leading to a different susceptibility for various pathogens.[71] The serotoxins secreted by S. aureus are able to penetrate the skin barrier and contribute to the persistence and exacerbation of allergic skin inflammation in atopic dermatitis. A recent systematic review suggests that there is no evidence that combined topical antibacterial and corticosteroid therapy are an effective strategy for all patients with atopic dermatitis to reduce the risk of secondary infections.[72] Prolonged antibiotic therapy may increase the prevalence of antibiotic-resistant strains of S. aureus.[73] As a result, in clinical practice, antibiotics are only advised in patients with atopic dermatitis with secondary bacterial infections.

Cutaneous dissemination of the herpes simplex virus on eczematous skin (ie, eczema herpeticum) is almost exclusively associated with atopic dermatitis.[74] The occurrence of eczema herpeticum in these patients is considered to be caused by a disruption of the skin barrier unmasking nectin-1, a desmosomal protein with a relevant entry receptor for herpes simplex virus, and an insufficient immune response due to the underlying predisposition to a T helper type 2 response.[75] These type 2 cytokines induce a rapid apoptosis of plasmacytoid dendritic cells and natural killer cells and down-regulate the generation of antimicrobial peptides.[74] The keystone of eczema herpeticum treatment is prompt systemic antiviral therapy, such as acyclovir, and strict follow up including eye examination and hospitalization if necessary.[74]

Malignancies

Uncertainty exists regarding the risk of cancer in patients with atopic dermatitis. It has been hypothesized that cancer risk is increased because the hyper reactive state of the immune system favors tumor onset or that cancer immunosurveillance may operate more efficiently in inflamed skin, decreasing the chance of aberrant cell proliferation. Evidence supporting the immunosurveillance theory has been reported for glioma and acute lymphoblastic leukemia (ALL). A meta-analysis of eight observational studies including a total of 3450 patients diagnosed with glioma, found a pooled relative risk for glioma of 0.69 (95% CI = 0.58 to 0.82) for patients with a history of eczema compared with patients without this condition.[76] Two large population-based case-control studies found a statistically significant reduced risk of between 30% to 50% for ALL in children with a history of eczema/atopic dermatitis, but this association was not confirmed in another study of 180 ALL cases.[77–79] It is unclear whether an atopic constitution or environmental factors that cause or exacerbate atopic dermatitis are responsible for the possible protective effect. Many methodological problems and possible sources of bias, including study designs, case definitions, recall bias, and the inability to analyze confounders and effect modifiers, cloud the issue.[78,80] Some therapies, such as phototherapy and cyclosporine, may increase the risk of cancers including skin cancers, as seen in patients with psoriasis, but no good, long-term, observational data are available in this patient population. Long-term safety studies of topical calcineurin inhibitors are also lacking.

VITILIGO

Vitiligo has frequently been described in association with autoimmune diseases, particularly autoimmune thyroid diseases like Graves' disease and autoimmune hypothyroidism.[81] In a retrospective study of 293 Korean patients with autoimmune thyroid disease, 6.8% had vitiligo compared with 0.9% of controls with non-autoimmune thyroid disease and 0.8% of the healthy controls.[82] In a German cohort of 321 patients with vitiligo, a high prevalence of autoimmune thyroiditis was detected.[83] Because vitiligo can precede thyroid disease by many years, some researchers suggest regular screening for thyroid dysfunction and thyroid related autoantibodies, but the prevalence of subclinical hypothyroidism is between 4% to 10% in those without a history of thyroid diseases, questioning the usefulness of this approach.[84–87] In addition to thyroid disease, vitiligo may co-exist with other autoimmune disease like type I diabetes mellitus, pernicious anemia, Addison's disease, alopecia areata, and celiac disease, but the epidemiologic evidence for these associations is weak.[84] Combinations of these diseases are described as autoimmune polyglandular syndromes. These genetic syndromes, especially type 1 and 3, in which autoantibodies are thought to be the cause of destruction of endocrine cells, are also associated with the presence of vitiligo. A genetic-linkage study identified a strong candidate gene, called NAPL1, contributing to a group of autoimmune and autoinflammatory diseases including vitiligo. This study demonstrated that DNA sequence variants in this region are associated with vitiligo alone, or with a more extended autoimmune phenotype, which can also comprise vitiligo.[88] Additional research is still essential on these associations and their frequency of occurrence, but informing and educating patients with regards to the signs and symptoms of these autoimmune diseases is advisable.

NONMELANOMA SKIN CANCER

Nonmelanoma skin cancer (NMSC) is the most common cancer in Caucasians and refers to

BCC and SCC. Increased childhood UV exposure is the most important risk factor of NMSC in predisposed individuals (eg, fair skin type, blond hair, and blue eyes). Recently, multiple studies have investigated comorbidities in patients with NMSC because NMSC is considered a proxy for high-UV exposure, which may relate to vitamin D levels that affect the development of several diseases and cancers (the so-called, "vitamin D hypothesis").[62,63] A population-based cohort study of nearly 27,000 patients with SCC showed a decreased risk of colorectal cancer of 19% to 36% compared with controls without NMSC. For cutaneous melanoma, which like BCC, is more strongly related to sunburns than cumulative sun exposure, an almost two folds increased risk of breast cancer was observed in women of 60 years and older.[89] Another international- cohort study that included more than 400,000 individuals with skin cancer, observed a significantly decreased prevalence of various internal solid cancers in patients with a prior NMSC, especially in sunny countries.[64] In contrast to the protective effects of NMSC, a recent large, Swedish study detected an increased total mortality among patients with SCC partly caused by an excess rate of deaths from cancers (SMR 2.17, 95% CI 2.08-2.26) and a small reduction in cancer mortality in BCC patients (SMR 0.95, 95% CI 0.96-0.98) compared with the general population.[90] Confounding factors, such as life-style (eg, diet habits and smoking status) and socioeconomic status, which are associated with developing NMSC and the risk of other cancers, may have affected the different study outcomes. In two large, prospective cohort studies of men and women in the United States, vitamin D intake was not related to BCC risk.[91] However, genetic studies suggest that vitamin D receptor polymorphisms may interact with nutritional vitamin D and affect the risk of NMSC and melanoma.[92–94]

The vitamin D hypothesis has raised a discussion about the benefits of UV exposure. However, 15 minutes of sun exposure on face and hands three times a week seems to be sufficient to maintain normal levels of vitamin D, suggesting that most people will spend enough time in the sun.[95] Future studies are needed to compare vitamin D levels in patients with NMSC and those without NMSC, and to further explain the observed differences.

HEALTH RELATED QUALITY OF LIFE AND DEPRESSION IN DERMATOLOGY

In general, psychodermatologic disorders are separated into psychiatric diseases that have a cutaneous association (eg, acne excoree and body dysmorphic disorder), and skin diseases that can be initiated or exacerbated by psychosocial stress or lead to a wide range of psychiatric disorders, including major depressive disorder, and even increased suicide risk.[96] A large group of dermatologic disorders are associated with having a major impact on HRQOL. Psychiatric disturbance and psychosocial impairment are reported in at least 30% of patients with dermatologic disorders.[97] In an Italian cross-sectional study of more than 2000 patients with a skin condition, 23% were considered to have psychiatric morbidity based on the General Health Questionnaire, and older women were especially at risk.[98] The impact of a disease on patients' lives did not correlate well with disease severity, and physicians are likely to underestimate the impact of the disease. The domains affected by dermatologic conditions differ between skin diseases. Inflammatory dermatoses have a larger impact on functional and physical domains, whereas vitiligo and alopecia areata may have a large effect on emotional well-being, and skin cancer affects anxiety and fear of recurrence.[99] These differences between diseases emphasize the need for selecting the most optimal HRQOL instruments for study goals and populations.[99]

In dermatology, the impact of psoriasis is probably the most studied. HRQOL impairment, assessed by the "SF-36 Health Survey," in patients with psoriasis is comparable to that of patients with chronic diseases such as cancer, arthritis, heart disease, and diabetes.[100] Compared with the general population, the prevalence of depression was significantly higher in patients with psoriasis.[101–103] A cross-sectional survey (response rate of 61%) noted depressive symptoms among 60% of the 2391 individuals with psoriasis. Lower educational levels, younger age, and the presence of itch were associated with reporting more depressive symptoms.[102,104,105] Data on the exact prevalence of depression among patients with psoriasis are not available, since different depression scoring methods or self reported data were used in the various studies on this association.

Higher levels of anxiety and depressive symptoms have also been reported in patients with atopic dermatitis, which may represent an underlying primary depressive disorder in some patients who have atopic dermatitis.[106–108] Consistent with findings in patients with psoriasis, the pruritus severity was also directly related to the presence of depressive symptoms among patients with atopic dermatitis.[109] A recent study suggested that the activation of the TNF-alpha system may contribute to the development of a depressive disorder. This hypothesis was based on an examination of the disease history of more than 1000 patients suffering from acute depressive episodes, where a history of depression was associated with a higher incidence of atopic eczema.[110] In patients with acute depression, the TNF-alpha levels and their soluble plasma receptor levels were also significantly elevated, suggesting a role for TNF-alpha in this association. In psoriasis, treatment with a TNF-alpha antagonist affected the presence of depression, which may have been related to a patients' decreased inflammatory state or improved HRQOL due to disease control.[111]

Physicians treating patients with a dermatologic disease should be alert to the impact of the disease on patients' lives, which may results in decreased HRQOL, feelings of stigmatization, or depressions. In conjunction to dermatologic care, psychological counseling or psychotropic medication may optimize the management of a subgroup of patients with chronic skin diseases. Moreover, a more holistic approach is likely to reduce the physical and emotional burden for patients, and increase satisfaction with care and treatment compliance.

REFERENCES

1. Feinstein A. The pretherapeutic classification of co-morbidity in chronic disease. J Chronic Dis 1970; 23:455–68.
2. Wikipedia. Comorbidity. Available at: http://en.wikipedia.org/wiki/Comorbidity. Last accessed 29 September 2008.
3. Chen T, Bertenthal D, Sahay A, et al. Predictors of skin-related quality of life after treatment of cutaneous basal cell carcinoma and squamous cell carcinoma. Arch Dermatol 2007;143:1386–92.
4. Christophers E. Comorbidities in psoriasis. Clin Dermatol 2007;25:529–34.
5. Gelfand JM, Gladman DD, Mease PJ, et al. Epidemiology of psoriatic arthritis in the population of the United States. J Am Acad Dermatol 2005;53:573–7.
6. Moll JM, Wright V. Psoriatic arthritis. Semin Arthritis Rheum 1973;3:55–78.
7. Taylor W, Gladman D, Helliwell P, et al. Classification criteria for psoriatic arthritis: development of new criteria from a large international study. Arthritis Rheum 2006;54:2665–73.
8. Finzi AF, Gibelli E. Psoriatic arthritis. Int J Dermatol 1991;30:1–7.
9. Rahman P, Gladman DD, Cook RJ, et al. Radiological assessment in psoriatic arthritis. Br J Rheumatol 1998;37:760–5.
10. Gladman DD, Mease PJ, Ritchlin CT, et al. Adalimumab for long-term treatment of psoriatic arthritis: forty-eight week data from the adalimumab effectiveness in psoriatic arthritis trial. Arthritis Rheum 2007;56:476–88.
11. Kavanaugh AF, Ritchlin CT. Systematic review of treatments for psoriatic arthritis: an evidence based approach and basis for treatment guidelines. J Rheumatol 2006;33:1417–21.
12. Krueger G, Ellis CN. Psoriasis–recent advances in understanding its pathogenesis and treatment. J Am Acad Dermatol 2005;53:S94–100.
13. Wakkee M, Thio HB, Prens EP, et al. Unfavorable cardiovascular risk profiles in untreated and treated psoriasis patients. Atherosclerosis 2007;190:1–9.
14. McDonald CJ, Calabresi P. Occlusive vascular disease in psoriatic patients. N Engl J Med 1973; 288:912.
15. Lindegard B. Diseases associated with psoriasis in a general population of 159,200 middle-aged, urban, native Swedes. Dermatologica 1986;172: 298–304.
16. Stern RS, Lange R. Cardiovascular disease, cancer, and cause of death in patients with psoriasis: 10 years prospective experience in a cohort of 1,380 patients. J Invest Dermatol 1988;91: 197–201.
17. Mallbris L, Akre O, Granath F, et al. Increased risk for cardiovascular mortality in psoriasis inpatients but not in outpatients. Eur J Epidemiol 2004;19: 225–30.
18. Sommer DM, Jenisch S, Suchan M, et al. Increased prevalence of the metabolic syndrome in patients with moderate to severe psoriasis. Arch Dermatol Res 2006;298:321–8.
19. Gisondi P, Tessari G, Conti A, et al. Prevalence of metabolic syndrome in patients with psoriasis: a hospital-based case-control study. Br J Dermatol 2007;157:68–73.
20. Gelfand JM, Neimann AL, Shin DB, et al. Risk of myocardial infarction in patients with psoriasis. JAMA 2006;296:1735–41.
21. Kaye JA, Li L, Jick SS, et al. Incidence of risk factors for myocardial infarction and other vascular diseases in patients with psoriasis. Br J Dermatol 2008;159:895–902.
22. Neimann AL, Shin DB, Wang X, et al. Prevalence of cardiovascular risk factors in patients with psoriasis. J Am Acad Dermatol 2006;55:829–35.
23. Setty AR, Curhan G, Choi HK, et al. Obesity, waist circumference, weight change, and the risk of psoriasis in women: Nurses' Health Study II. Arch Intern Med 2007;167:1670–5.
24. Naldi L, Chatenoud L, Linder D, et al. Cigarette smoking, body mass index, and stressful life events as risk factors for psoriasis: results from an Italian case-control study. J Invest Dermatol 2005;125:61–7.
25. Brauchli YB, Jick SS, Curtin F, et al. Association between beta-blockers, other antihypertensive

drugs and psoriasis: population-based case-control study. Br J Dermatol 2008;158:1299–307.

26. Wakkee M, van der Linden M, Nijsten T, et al. Psoriasis appears not to be directly related with using cardiovascular and antidiabetic drugs. J Invest Dermatol 2008;128:1299–307.

27. Kimball AB, Gladman D, Gelfand JM, et al. National Psoriasis Foundation clinical consensus on psoriasis comorbidities and recommendations for screening. J Am Acad Dermatol 2008;58:1031–42.

28. Margolis D, Bilker W, Hennessy S, et al. The risk of malignancy associated with psoriasis. Arch Dermatol 2001;137:778–83.

29. Frentz G, Olsen JH. Malignant tumours and psoriasis: a follow-up study. Br J Dermatol 1999;140:237–42.

30. Boffetta P, Gridley G, Lindelof B, et al. Cancer risk in a population-based cohort of patients hospitalized for psoriasis in Sweden. J Invest Dermatol 2001;117:1531–7.

31. Marcil I, Stern RS. Squamous-cell cancer of the skin in patients given PUVA and cyclosporine: nested cohort crossover study. Lancet 2001;358:1042–5.

32. Stern RS. The risk of melanoma in association with long-term exposure to PUVA. J Am Acad Dermatol 2001;44:755–61.

33. Roelofzen JH, Aben KK, van der Valk PG, et al. Coal tar in dermatology. J Dermatolog Treat 2007;18:329–34.

34. Naldi L, Parazzini F, Brevi A, et al. Family history, smoking habits, alcohol consumption and risk of psoriasis. Br J Dermatol 1992;127:212–7.

35. Poikolainen K, Reunala T, Karvonen J, et al. Alcohol intake: a risk factor for psoriasis in young and middle aged men? BMJ 1990;300:780–3.

36. Gelfand JM, Berlin J, Van Voorhees A, et al. Lymphoma rates are low but increased in patients with psoriasis: results from a population-based cohort study in the United Kingdom. Arch Dermatol 2003;139:1425–9.

37. Gelfand JM, Shin DB, Neimann AL, et al. The risk of lymphoma in patients with psoriasis. J Invest Dermatol 2006;126:2194–201.

38. Stern RS. Lymphoma risk in psoriasis: results of the PUVA follow-up study. Arch Dermatol 2006;142:1132–5.

39. Paul CF, Ho VC, McGeown C, et al. Risk of malignancies in psoriasis patients treated with cyclosporine: a 5 y cohort study. J Invest Dermatol 2003;120:211–6.

40. Bongartz T, Sutton AJ, Sweeting MJ, et al. Anti-TNF antibody therapy in rheumatoid arthritis and the risk of serious infections and malignancies: systematic review and meta-analysis of rare harmful effects in randomized controlled trials. JAMA 2006;295:2275–85.

41. Norrlind R. The significance of infections in the origination of psoriasis. Acta Rheumatol Scand 1955;1:135–44.

42. Gudjonsson JE, Thorarinsson AM, Sigurgeirsson B, et al. Streptococcal throat infections and exacerbation of chronic plaque psoriasis: a prospective study. Br J Dermatol 2003;149:530–4.

43. Tomi NS, Kranke B, Aberer E, et al. Staphylococcal toxins in patients with psoriasis, atopic dermatitis, and erythroderma, and in healthy control subjects. J Am Acad Dermatol 2005;53:67–72.

44. Henseler T, Christophers E. Disease concomitance in psoriasis. J Am Acad Dermatol 1995;32:982–6.

45. Harder J, Bartels J, Christophers E, et al. A peptide antibiotic from human skin. Nature 1997;387:861.

46. Lande R, Gregorio J, Facchinetti V, et al. Plasmacytoid dendritic cells sense self-DNA coupled with antimicrobial peptide. Nature 2007;449:564–9.

47. Hollox EJ, Huffmeier U, Zeeuwen PL, et al. Psoriasis is associated with increased beta-defensin genomic copy number. Nat Genet 2008;40:23–5.

48. Drancourt M, Argenson JN, Tissot Dupont H, et al. Psoriasis is a risk factor for hip-prosthesis infection. Eur J Epidemiol 1997;13:205–7.

49. Sadick NS, McNutt NS, Kaplan MH, et al. Papulosquamous dermatoses of AIDS. J Am Acad Dermatol 1990;22:1270–7.

50. Patel RV, Weinberg JM. Psoriasis in the patient with human immunodeficiency virus, part 1: review of pathogenesis. Cutis 2008;82:117–22.

51. Zhang XJ, Zhang AP, Yang S, et al. Association of HLA class I alleles with psoriasis vulgaris in southeastern Chinese Hans. J Dermatol Sci 2003;33:1–6.

52. Goh BK, Chan RK, Sen P, et al. Spectrum of skin disorders in human immunodeficiency virus-infected patients in Singapore and the relationship to CD4 lymphocyte counts. Int J Dermatol 2007;46:695–9.

53. Smith JD, Knox JM. Psoriasis, methotrexate and tuberculosis. Br J Dermatol 1971;84:590–3.

54. Vachharajani TJ, Oza UG, Phadke AG, et al. Tuberculosis in renal transplant recipients: rifampicin sparing treatment protocol. Int Urol Nephrol 2002;34:551–3.

55. Kroesen S, Widmer AF, Tyndall A, et al. Serious bacterial infections in patients with rheumatoid arthritis under anti-TNF-alpha therapy. Rheumatology (Oxford) 2003;42:617–21.

56. Lebwohl M, Bagel J, Gelfand JM, et al. From the Medical Board of the National Psoriasis Foundation: monitoring and vaccinations in patients treated with biologics for psoriasis. J Am Acad Dermatol 2008;58:94–105.

57. Lee FI, Bellary SV, Francis C, et al. Increased occurrence of psoriasis in patients with Crohn's disease and their relatives. Am J Gastroenterol 1990;85:962–3.

58. Kia KF, Nair RP, Ike RW, et al. Prevalence of anti-gliadin antibodies in patients with psoriasis is not elevated compared with controls. Am J Clin Dermatol 2007;8:301–5.

59. Michaelsson G, Gerden B, Ottosson M, et al. Patients with psoriasis often have increased serum levels of IgA antibodies to gliadin. Br J Dermatol 1993;129:667–73.

60. Damasiewicz-Bodzek A, Wielkoszynski T. Serologic markers of celiac disease in psoriatic patients. J Eur Acad Dermatol Venereol 2008;22:1055–61.

61. Dreiher J, Weitzman D, Shapiro J, et al. Psoriasis and chronic obstructive pulmonary disease: a case-control study. Br J Dermatol 2008;159: 956–60.

62. Spergel JM, Paller AS. Atopic dermatitis and the atopic march. J Allergy Clin Immunol 2003;112: S118–27.

63. Burrows B, Martinez FD, Halonen M, et al. Association of asthma with serum IgE levels and skin-test reactivity to allergens. N Engl J Med 1989; 320:271–7.

64. Wuthrich B. Serum IgE in atopic dermatitis: relationship to severity of cutaneous involvement and course of disease as well as coexistence of atopic respiratory diseases. Clin Allergy 1978;8:241–8.

65. Eichenfield LF, Hanifin JM, Beck LA, et al. Atopic dermatitis and asthma: parallels in the evolution of treatment. Pediatrics 2003;111:608–16.

66. Kondo H, Ichikawa Y, Imokawa G, et al. Percutaneous sensitization with allergens through barrier-disrupted skin elicits a Th2-dominant cytokine response. Eur J Immunol 1998;28:769–79.

67. Warner JO. A double-blinded, randomized, placebo-controlled trial of cetirizine in preventing the onset of asthma in children with atopic dermatitis: 18 months' treatment and 18 months' post-treatment follow-up. J Allergy Clin Immunol 2001; 108:929–37.

68. Bustos GJ, Bustos D, Bustos GJ, et al. Prevention of asthma with ketotifen in preasthmatic children: a three-year follow-up study. Clin Exp Allergy 1995;25:568–73.

69. Cole GW, Silverberg NL. The adherence of staphylococcus aureus to human corneocytes. Arch Dermatol 1986;122:166–9.

70. Ong PY, Ohtake T, Brandt C, et al. Endogenous antimicrobial peptides and skin infections in atopic dermatitis. N Engl J Med 2002;347: 1151–60.

71. Zeeuwen PL, de Jongh GJ, Rodijk-Olthuis D, et al. Genetically programmed differences in epidermal host defense between psoriasis and atopic dermatitis patients. PLoS ONE 2008;3:e2301.

72. Birnie AJ, Bath-Hextall F, Ravenscroft JC, et al. Interventions to reduce staphylococcus aureus in the management of atopic eczema. Cochrane Database Syst Rev 2008;3:CD003871.

73. Lin YT, Wang CT, Chiang BL, et al. Role of bacterial pathogens in atopic dermatitis. Clin Rev Allergy Immunol 2007;33:167–77.

74. Wollenberg A, Klein E. Current aspects of innate and adaptive immunity in atopic dermatitis. Clin Rev Allergy Immunol 2007;33:35–44.

75. Yoon M, Spear PG. Disruption of adherens junctions liberates nectin-1 to serve as receptor for herpes simplex virus and pseudorabies virus entry. J Virol 2002;76:7203–8.

76. Linos E, Raine T, Alonso A, et al. Atopy and risk of brain tumors: a meta-analysis. J Natl Cancer Inst 2007;99:1544–50.

77. Wen W, Shu XO, Linet MS, et al. Allergic disorders and the risk of childhood acute lymphoblastic leukemia (United States). Cancer Causes Control 2000;11:303–7.

78. Spector L, Groves F, DeStefano F, et al. Medically recorded allergies and the risk of childhood acute lymphoblastic leukaemia. Eur J Cancer 2004;40: 579–84.

79. Schuz J, Morgan G, Bohler E, et al. Atopic disease and childhood acute lymphoblastic leukemia. Int J Cancer 2003;105:255–60.

80. Wang H, Diepgen TL. Is atopy a protective or a risk factor for cancer? A review of epidemiological studies. Allergy 2005;60:1098–111.

81. Alkhateeb A, Fain PR, Thody A, et al. Epidemiology of vitiligo and associated autoimmune diseases in Caucasian probands and their families. Pigment Cell Res 2003;16:208–14.

82. Shong YK, Kim JA. Vitiligo in autoimmune thyroid disease. Thyroid 1991;3:89–91.

83. Schallreuter KU, Lemke R, Brandt O, et al. Vitiligo and other diseases: coexistence or true association? Hamburg study on 321 patients. Dermatology 1994;188:269–75.

84. Amerio P, Tracanna M, De Remigis P, et al. Vitiligo associated with other autoimmune diseases: polyglandular autoimmune syndrome types 3B+C and 4. Clin Exp Dermatol 2006;31:746–9.

85. Dittmar M, Kahaly GJ. Polyglandular autoimmune syndromes: immunogenetics and long-term follow-up. J Clin Endocrinol Metab 2003;88: 2983–92.

86. Canaris GJ, Manowitz NR, Mayor G, et al. The Colorado thyroid disease prevalence study. Arch Intern Med 2000;160:526–34.

87. Hollowell JG, Staehling NW, Flanders WD, et al. Serum TSH, T(4), and thyroid antibodies in the United States population (1988 to 1994): National Health and Nutrition Examination Survey (NHANES III). J Clin Endocrinol Metab 2002;87: 489–99.

88. Jin Y, Mailloux CM, Gowan K, et al. NALP1 in viti-ligo-associated multiple autoimmune disease. N Engl J Med 2007;356:1216–25.

89. Soerjomataram I, Louwman WJ, Lemmens VE, et al. Are patients with skin cancer at lower risk of developing colorectal or breast cancer? Am J Epidemiol 2008;167:1421–9.

90. Jensen AO, Bautz A, Olesen AB, et al. Mortality in Danish patients with nonmelanoma skin cancer, 1978–2001. Br J Dermatol 2008;159:419–25.

91. Hunter DJ, Colditz GA, Stampfer MJ, et al. Diet and risk of basal cell carcinoma of the skin in a prospective cohort of women. Ann Epidemiol 1992;2:231–9.

92. Han J, Colditz GA, Hunter DJ, et al. Polymorphisms in the MTHFR and VDR genes and skin cancer risk. Carcinogenesis 2007;28:390–7.

93. Li C, Liu Z, Zhang Z, et al. Genetic variants of the vitamin D receptor gene alter risk of cutaneous melanoma. J Invest Dermatol 2007;127:276–80.

94. Bikle DD. Vitamin D receptor, UVR, and skin cancer: a potential protective mechanism. J Invest Dermatol 2008;128:2357–61.

95. Holick MF. McCollum Award Lecture, 1994: vitamin D–new horizons for the 21st century. Am J Clin Nutr 1994;60:619–30.

96. Cotterill JA, Cunliffe WJ. Suicide in dermatological patients. Br J Dermatol 1997;137:246–50.

97. Fried RG, Gupta MA, Gupta AK, et al. Depression and skin disease. Dermatol Clin 2005;23:657–64.

98. Sampogna F, Picardi A, Chren MM, et al. Association between poorer quality of life and psychiatric morbidity in patients with different dermatological conditions. Psychosom Med 2004;66:620–4.

99. Both H, Essink-Bot ML, Busschbach J, et al. Critical review of generic and dermatology-specific health-related quality of life instruments. J Invest Dermatol 2007;127:2726–39.

100. Rapp SR, Feldman SR, Exum ML, et al. Psoriasis causes as much disability as other major medical diseases. J Am Acad Dermatol 1999;41:401–7.

101. Sharma N, Koranne RV, Singh RK, et al. Psychiatric morbidity in psoriasis and vitiligo: a comparative study. J Dermatol 2001;28:419–23.

102. Esposito M, Saraceno R, Giunta A, et al. An Italian study on psoriasis and depression. Dermatology 2006;212:123–7.

103. Akay A, Pekcanlar A, Bozdag KE, et al. Assessment of depression in subjects with psoriasis vulgaris and lichen planus. J Eur Acad Dermatol Venereol 2002;16:347–52.

104. Gupta MA, Gupta AK, Watteel GN, et al. Early onset (< 40 years age) psoriasis is comorbid with greater psychopathology than late onset psoriasis: a study of 137 patients. Acta Derm Venereol 1996; 76:464–6.

105. Gupta MA, Gupta AK, Kirkby S, et al. Pruritus in psoriasis. A prospective study of some psychiatric and dermatologic correlates. Arch Dermatol 1988; 124:1052–7.

106. Ahmar H, Kurban AK. Psychological profile of patients with atopic dermatitis. Br J Dermatol 1976;95:373–7.

107. Linnet J, Jemec GB. An assessment of anxiety and dermatology life quality in patients with atopic dermatitis. Br J Dermatol 1999;140:268–72.

108. Hashiro M, Okumura M. Anxiety, depression and psychosomatic symptoms in patients with atopic dermatitis: comparison with normal controls and among groups of different degrees of severity. J Dermatol Sci 1997;14:63–7.

109. Gupta MA, Gupta AK, Schork NJ, et al. Depression modulates pruritus perception: a study of pruritus in psoriasis, atopic dermatitis, and chronic idiopathic urticaria. Psychosom Med 1994;56:36–40.

110. Himmerich H, Fulda S, Linseisen J, et al. Depression, comorbidities and the TNF-alpha system. Eur Psychiatry 2008;23:421–9.

111. Tyring S, Gottlieb A, Papp K, et al. Etanercept and clinical outcomes, fatigue, and depression in psoriasis: double-blind placebo-controlled randomised phase III trial. Lancet 2006;367:29–35.

The Benefits and Risks of Ultraviolet Tanning and Its Alternatives: The Role of Prudent Sun Exposure

Raja K. Sivamani, MS[a], Lori A. Crane, PhD, MPH[b,c],
Robert P. Dellavalle, MD, PhD, MSPH[b,d,e,*]

KEYWORDS

- Tanning • Ultraviolet light • Health • Benefits • Risks
- Sun • Vitamin D

Deliberate tanning is a common practice among light-skinned individuals in Europe and United States.[1–4] Many health benefits and risks have been attributed to ultraviolet (UV) exposure and tanning. This article discusses these claims in light of the growing indoor UV and non-UV tanning industries.

HEALTH BENEFITS

Several health benefit claims, such as improved appearance, enhanced mood, and increased vitamin D levels, have been attributed to tanning. Furthermore, the Indoor Tanning Association claims, "catching some rays may lengthen your life."[5]

Exposure to sunlight has been linked to improved energy and elevated mood. The belief that people look better with a tan may partially explain this phenomenon. A report on the tanning attitudes of young adults found that 81% of individuals in 2007 believed that a tan improved appearance, whereas only 58% of individuals in 1968 held the same belief.[6] Individuals who have seasonal affective disorder report improved mood status when exposed to sunlight[7] and to frequent tanning.[8] Although early studies suggested that mood elevation was linked to increased endorphin levels,[9] subsequent studies have not found such a correlation.[10–12]

The Indoor Tanning Association claims that a base tan can act as "the body's natural protection against sunburn."[5] UV-induced tans offer a sun protection factor of 3 to 4,[13,14] but additional changes besides hyperpigmentation, such as epidermal hyperplasia, likely play a role in UV-induced photoprotection. Although a sun protection factor of 3 to 4 does protect from sunburn, only approximately 65% of the erythema induced by UV radiation is blocked.[15] Therefore, a base tan does not provide adequate protection, and

Supported by University of Colorado Denver, School of Medicine, Colorado Health Informatics Collaboration interdisciplinary academic enrichment funds (RPD) and National Cancer Institute grants RO1-CA74592 (LAC) and K-07 CA92550 (RPD).

a University of California, Davis, School of Medicine, 4610 X Street, Sacramento, CA 95817, USA
b Colorado School of Public Health, 4200 E. Ninth Avenue, Campus Box B119, Denver, CO 80262, USA
c University of Colorado at Denver Health Sciences Center, 4200 East Ninth Avenue, Campus Box B119, Denver, CO 80262, USA
d Dermatology Service, Department of Veterans Affairs Medical Center, 1055 Clermont Street, Mail Code 165, Denver, CO 80220, USA
e Department of Dermatology, University of Colorado Denver, School of Medicine, Aurora, CO 80045, USA
* Corresponding author. Colorado School of Public Health, 13001 E. 17th Place, Campus Box B119, Aurora, CO, 80045.
E-mail address: robert.dellavalle@ucdenver.edu (R.P. Dellavalle).

Dermatol Clin 27 (2009) 149–154
doi:10.1016/j.det.2008.11.008
0733-8635/08/$ – see front matter. Published by Elsevier Inc.

derm.theclinics.com

appropriate clothing, the proper use of sunscreens, and prudent sun exposure remain essential for sunburn prevention.

VITAMIN D PRODUCTION

Sunlight contains UV-B, which induces the skin to synthesize previtamin D3. Healthy individuals have seasonal variations in their vitamin D levels[16,17] and may become vitamin D deficient during winter.[17] Lower vitamin D levels are associated with increased risk for several types of cancer, heart disease, and bone disease.[18–23] Vitamin D deficiency also may play a role in autoimmune disease.[24]

The Indoor Tanning Association highlights "new research on how sunshine decreases infection,"[5] including a West African case-control study in which more patients who had tuberculosis than controls had low levels of vitamin D (hypovitaminosis defined as 25-hydroxyvitamin D3 (25(OH)D3) $\leq$ 75 nmol/L) (46% versus 39%) (relative risk [RR] 1.18; 95% CI, 1.01–1.38).[25] Even lower levels of vitamin D (vitamin D deficiency defined as 25(OH)D3 $\leq$ 50 nmol/L), however, were less common among patients who had tuberculosis than controls (8.5% versus 13.2%) (RR 0.65; 95% CI, 0.43–0.98). The causal relation of these associations is unknown.

The current recommendation for daily intake of vitamin D is 400 to 600 IU, but the required daily intake likely should be increased to 800 to 2000 IU[26,27] to maintain blood levels of 25-hydroxyvitamin D (25(OH)D) greater than 75 nmol/L. Although UV tanning leads to the endogenous synthesis of previtamin D3, several studies in human skin have shown that total previtamin D3 production in the skin plateaus with exposure time.[28] Further increases in UV exposure do not increase the total amount of previtamin D3. A moderate amount of sun exposure to the hands, face, and arms every other day produces enough cutaneous previtamin D3 to meet daily requirements in light-skinned persons, even if the daily requirements are increased to 1000 IU.[29,30] Calculations demonstrate that individuals who have lighter skin (types I–III) need 5 to 20 minutes of sun exposure depending on season. These recommendations also apply at higher latitudes where sun-induced vitamin D synthesis is less efficient.[30] Moderate sun exposure is as efficient as prolonged sun exposure for previtamin D production. Sunlight exposure as the only source of vitamin D may be impractical, however, in cold weather and for those who have darker skin types.[30] Therefore, moderate sunlight exposure should be considered in combination with a diet fortified with vitamin D for optimal vitamin D status.

In one study, UV tanners had twice the 25(OH)D levels as nontanners,[31] even after controlling for variations in ethnicity between the two groups.[32] The decreased vitamin D status of the nontanners, however, may be a reflection of inadequate daily recommendations, because the current recommended daily allowance for vitamin D may be insufficient.[26,27] Future studies are necessary to determine whether or not increased daily recommendations and intake of vitamin D would diminish the discrepancy between tanners and nontanners.

HEALTH RISKS

Although UV radiation promotes skin malignancies, such as basal cell carcinoma (BCC), squamous cell carcinoma (SCC), and melanoma, the most serious of these cancers, the association for each type of skin cancer differs.[33] Intermittent sun exposure and sunburns are associated positively with melanoma,[34,35] whereas chronic sun exposure is not.[35] A weak association and dose-response relationship exists between sunbed use and melanoma,[36] including a doubling of the risk for developing melanoma in individuals who start using tanning beds before age 35.[36] Studies may be limited by recall bias, because individuals who develop melanoma are more likely to recall a history of increased sun exposure and sunburns.[34,35] Melanoma also is strongly associated with immigration during childhood from low to high UV radiation geographic locations.[37] This ecologic study did not depend on personal recall of sun exposure and, therefore, is less susceptible to recall bias, but the role of childhood sunburns was not addressed specifically.

SCC and BCC demonstrate varying relationships between UV exposure from sunlight and UV tanning beds. A detailed review of case-control studies showed that cumulative sun exposure was associated with BCCs and SCCs, whereas intermittent sun exposure was associated with only BCCs.[38] A history of sunburn increased the risk for developing BCCs and SCCs. Childhood sunburns were associated with SCCs, whereas sunburns at any age were associated with BCCs.[38] Indoor tanning was associated with SCC but not BCCs.[36]

Frequent exposure to sunlight also accelerates skin aging. Much of this aging process has been attributed to UV exposure[39] and subsequent free radical generation,[40] with infrared radiation playing an important role. Infrared radiation likely promotes photoaging by inducing the breakdown of collagen and increasing the presence of reactive oxygen species.[41,42] Physical sun-blocking agents, such as titanium dioxide, block infrared radiation,[41] but most chemical-based sunblocks were developed for UV, not infrared, photoprotection.

ROLE OF INDOOR TANNING

Indoor tanning is widespread in the United States: 8% to 20% of adults[43] and 7% to 35% of teens[44] have engaged in indoor tanning as have up to 48% of 18- to 19-year-old white women.[45] Indoor tanning increases the risk for skin cancer,[36,46,47] augments the risk for sunburn, and accelerates photoaging.[39] Indoor tanning practices are greatly influenced by parental acceptance and peer participation.[48,49] Indoor tanners also spend more time outdoors,[43] increasing their UV exposure and further elevating their risks for sunburns and skin cancers. Young white women are cosmetically and socially motivated to tan.[50] Dark-skinned and elderly populations who are at the highest risk for vitamin D deficiency[51] and would benefit the most from sun exposure are the least likely to engage in indoor or outdoor tanning. Many teens tan indoors,[44,48] and many indoor tanning advertisements specifically target this population.[52,53] Because tanning may be addictive,[54,55] and because it promotes premature skin aging and skin cancer,[36] many states have enacted laws to limit teen access to indoor tanning.[56] Although these laws reduce indoor tanning among teens,[53] they are poorly enforced.[57,58]

SUNLESS TANNING

An alternative to UV tanning is sunless tanning. Currently marketed sunless tanning agents include spray-on tans and sunless tanning lotions. These products contain dihydroxyacetone (DHA), which reacts with the amino groups in the stratum corneum to stain the skin brown. Although DHA protects against UV-A[59] and UV-B,[60] this protection is transient and inadequate. Therefore, other protective measures, such as clothing and sunscreen use, are necessary for sunburn protection. People using sunless tanning products were more likely to have had sunburn in the past year.[61] The beliefs and the temporal relationship regarding sunburn and sunless tanner use, however, deserve further study. (Eg, How often is sunless tanning a protective response because of past sunburn? How often does sunburn result from a false sense of photoprotection ascribed to a sunless tan?) DHA may temporarily increase the formation of UV radiation-induced reactive oxygen species for the first 24 hours after application,[62] leading to acceleration of sun-induced damage. Therefore, minimization of sun and UV exposure after application of DHA is advised during the first 24 hours after application.

People who rely solely on sunless tanning products exhibit better sun protection habits than those who tan indoors, those who use indoor and sunless tanning products, and those who refrain from tanning.[63] Sunscreen and protective clothing use is increased among exclusively sunless tanners. This contradicts earlier findings that associated sunless tanning with sunburn.[61] The earlier study did not examine, however, the temporal relationship between sunburn and sunless tanning. The study also did not differentiate between exclusively sunless tanners and those who used both sunless tanning and indoor tanning, which can confound whether or not the increased sunburns were the result of sunless tanning or indoor tanning habits. A prospective study of exclusively sunless tanners would lead to better understanding of how sunless tanning and sunburns are associated.

DHA-based sunless tanning agents have several drawbacks. The effect is temporary, the resulting skin color can look unnatural, and there is an increased risk for sun-induced damage within 24 hours of application.[62] The development of a new class of agents that enhance melanin production in the skin may address these concerns. Although no products currently are on the market, several possibilities are under research. Topical agents that activate the p53 cascade,[64] the β_2-adrenergic receptor and cyclic AMP–dependant pathways,[65,66] the melanocortin 1 receptor,[66] and the topical application of T-oligos[67] may hold the key to successful sunless tanning. A topical method to induce melanogenesis has many exciting possibilities and requires more research. Such products may induce a more natural-looking tan and make sunless tanning more desirable. These new agents may activate the body's natural tanning physiology while avoiding the drawbacks of UV damage.

SUMMARY

Sun exposure is beneficial in moderation but can be harmful in excess. Sun exposure guidance should be tailored to individual patients. Individual factors, such as skin type, past history of skin cancers, and concurrent medical conditions, should influence counseling practices. Tanning is achieved primarily through the overexposure of skin to UV radiation and is most prevalent among lighter-skinned populations. In these populations, UV tanning may not offer any benefit over moderate sun exposure to offset elevated skin cancer and photoaging risk. Sun exposure should not be used as an alternative but as an adjunct to a diet fortified with vitamin D. Sunless tanning products may serve as a sensible, safer alternative for those who desire tanned skin. The use of sunscreens, preferably with broad coverage against UV-A, UV-B, and infrared radiation, are essential for tanners who have prolonged UV and sunlight exposure.Tanners should be educated, however, that although sunscreens prevent sunburn and reduce the risk for SCC,[68] they do not seem to reduce the risk for the development of BCC[68] or melanoma.[69] Therefore, prudent sun exposure is paramount.

ACKNOWLEDGMENTS

The authors thank Kristine Busse and Adam Asarch for critical review of this manuscript.

REFERENCES

1. Melia J, Bulman A. Sunburn and tanning in a British population. J Public Health Med 1995;17(2):223–9.
2. Boldeman C, Branstrom R, Dal H, et al. Tanning habits and sunburn in a Swedish population age 13–50 years. Eur J Cancer 2001;37(18):2441–8.
3. Robinson JK, Rademaker AW, Sylvester JA, et al. Summer sun exposure: knowledge, attitudes, and behaviors of midwest adolescents. Prev Med 1997;26(3):364–72.
4. Fitzpatrick TB. The validity and practicality of sun-reactive skin types I through VI. Arch Dermatol 1988;124(6):869–71.
5. Website. Available at: http://www.theita.com. Accessed January 30, 2009.
6. Robinson JK, Kim J, Rosenbaum S, et al. Indoor tanning knowledge, attitudes, and behavior among young adults from 1988–2007. Arch Dermatol 2008;144(4):484–8.
7. Wirz-Justice A, Graw P, Krauchi K, et al. 'Natural' light treatment of seasonal affective disorder. J Affect Disord 1996;37(2–3):109–20.
8. Hillhouse J, Stapleton J, Turrisi R. Association of frequent indoor UV tanning with seasonal affective disorder. Arch Dermatol 2005;141(11):1465.
9. Levins PC, Carr DB, Fisher JE, et al. Plasma beta-endorphin and beta-lipoprotein response to ultraviolet radiation. Lancet 1983;2(8342):166.
10. Gambichler T, Bader A, Vojvodic M, et al. Plasma levels of opioid peptides after sunbed exposures. Br J Dermatol 2002;147(6):1207–11.
11. Kaur M, Liguori A, Fleischer AB Jr, et al. Plasma beta-endorphin levels in frequent and infrequent tanners before and after ultraviolet and non-ultraviolet stimuli. J Am Acad Dermatol 2006;54(5):919–20.
12. Wintzen M, Ostijn DM, Polderman MC, et al. Total body exposure to ultraviolet radiation does not influence plasma levels of immunoreactive beta-endorphin in man. Photodermatol Photoimmunol Photomed 2001;17(6):256–60.
13. Nonaka S, Kaidbey KH, Kligman AM. Photoprotective adaptation. Some quantitative aspects. Arch Dermatol 1984;120(5):609–12.
14. Cripps DJ. Natural and artificial photoprotection. J Invest Dermatol 1981;77(1):154–7.
15. Nash JF, Tanner PR, Matts PJ. Ultraviolet A radiation: testing and labeling for sunscreen products. Dermatol Clin 2006;24(1):63–74.
16. Moan J, Porojnicu AC, Dahlback A, et al. Addressing the health benefits and risks, involving vitamin D or skin cancer, of increased sun exposure. Proc Natl Acad Sci U S A 2008;105(2):668–73.
17. Tangpricha V, Pearce EN, Chen TC, et al. Vitamin D insufficiency among free-living healthy young adults. Am J Med 2002;112(8):659–62.
18. Giovannucci E. Epidemiological evidence for vitamin D and colorectal cancer. J Bone Miner Res 2007;22(s2):V81–5.
19. Mitka M. Vitamin D deficits may affect heart health. JAMA 2008;299(7):753–4.
20. Wang TJ, Pencina MJ, Booth SL, et al. Vitamin D deficiency and risk of cardiovascular disease. Circulation 2008;117(4):503–11.
21. Cranney A, Horsley T, O'Donnell S, et al. Effectiveness and safety of vitamin D in relation to bone health. Evid Rep Technol Assess (Full Rep) 2007;158:1–235.
22. Li H, Stampfer MJ, Hollis JB, et al. A prospective study of plasma vitamin D metabolites, vitamin D receptor polymorphisms, and prostate cancer. PLoS Med 2007;4(3):e103.
23. Dobnig H, Pilz S, Scharnagl H, et al. Independent association of low serum 25-hydroxyvitamin D and 1,25-dihydroxyvitamin D levels with all-cause and cardiovascular mortality. Arch Intern Med 2008;168(12):1340–9.
24. Lips P. Vitamin D physiology. Prog Biophys Mol Biol 2006;92(1):4–8.
25. Wejse C, Olesen R, Rabna P, et al. Serum 25-hydroxyvitamin D in a West African population of tuberculosis patients and unmatched healthy controls. Am J Clin Nutr 2007;86(5):1376–83.
26. Heaney RP. The vitamin D requirement in health and disease. J Steroid Biochem Mol Biol 2005;97(1–2):13–9.
27. Holick MF, Chen TC. Vitamin D deficiency: a worldwide problem with health consequences. Am J Clin Nutr 2008;87(4):1080S–6S.
28. Holick MF, MacLaughlin JA, Doppelt SH. Regulation of cutaneous previtamin D3 photosynthesis in man: skin pigment is not an essential regulator. Science 1981;211(4482):590–3.
29. Webb AR, Engelsen O. Ultraviolet exposure scenarios: risks of erythema from recommendations on cutaneous vitamin D synthesis. Adv Exp Med Biol 2008;624:72–85.

30. Webb AR, Engelsen O. Calculated ultraviolet expo-sure levels for a healthy vitamin D status. Photochem Photobiol 2006;82(6):1697–703.

31. Tangpricha V, Turner A, Spina C, et al. Tanning is associated with optimal vitamin D status (serum 25-hydroxyvitamin D concentration) and higher bone mineral density. Am J Clin Nutr 2004;80(6):1645–9.

32. Holick MF, Tangpricha V. Reply to MA Weinstock and D Lazovich. Am J Clin Nutr 2005;82(3):707–8.

33. Rigel DS. Cutaneous ultraviolet exposure and its relationship to the development of skin cancer. J Am Acad Dermatol 2008;58(5, Suppl2):S129–32.

34. Elwood JM. Melanoma and sun exposure. Semin Oncol 1996;23(6):650–66.

35. Gandini S, Sera F, Cattaruzza MS, et al. Meta-analy-sis of risk factors for cutaneous melanoma: II. Sun exposure. Eur J Cancer 2005;41(1):45–60.

36. International Agency for Research on Cancer Work-ing Group on Artificial Ultraviolet (UV) Light and Skin Cancer. The association of use of sunbeds with cu-taneous malignant melanoma and other skin can-cers: a systematic review. Int J Cancer 2007; 120(5):1116–22.

37. Whiteman DC, Whiteman CA, Green AC. Childhood sun exposure as a risk factor for melanoma: a sys-tematic review of epidemiologic studies. Cancer Causes Control 2001;12(1):69–82.

38. Almahroos M, Kurban AK. Ultraviolet carcinogenesis in nonmelanoma skin cancer part II: review and update on epidemiologic correlations. Skinmed 2004;3(3):132–9.

39. Pierard GE. Ageing in the sun parlour. Int J Cosmet Sci 1998;20(4):251–9.

40. Wenk J, Brenneisen P, Meewes C, et al. UV-induced oxidative stress and photoaging. Curr Probl Derma-tol 2001;29:83–94.

41. Schroeder P, Haendeler J, Krutmann J. The role of near infrared radiation in photoaging of the skin. Exp Gerontol 2008;43(7):629–32.

42. Schroeder P, Lademann J, Darvin ME, et al. Infrared radiation-induced matrix metalloproteinase in hu-man skin: implications for protection. J Invest Der-matol 2008;128(10):2491–7.

43. Heckman CJ, Coups EJ, Manne SL. Prevalence and correlates of indoor tanning among US adults. J Am Acad Dermatol 2008;58(5):769–80.

44. Geller AC, Colditz G, Oliveria S, et al. Use of sun-screen, sunburning rates, and tanning bed use among more than 10 000 US children and adoles-cents. Pediatrics 2002;109(6):1009–14.

45. Demko CA, Borawski EA, Debanne SM, et al. Use of indoor tanning facilities by white adolescents in the United States. Arch Pediatr Adolesc Med 2003; 157(9):854–60.

46. Swerdlow AJ, English JS, MacKie RM, et al. Fluores-cent lights, ultraviolet lamps, and risk of cutaneous melanoma. BMJ 1988;297(6649):647–50.

47. Ting W, Schultz K, Cac NN, et al. Tanning bed expo-sure increases the risk of malignant melanoma. Int J Dermatol 2007;46(12):1253–7.

48. Cokkinides VE, Weinstock MA, O'Connell MC, et al. Use of indoor tanning sunlamps by US youth, ages 11–18 years, and by their parent or guardian care-givers: prevalence and correlates. Pediatrics 2002; 109(6):1124–30.

49. Hoerster KD, Mayer JA, Woodruff SI, et al. The influ-ence of parents and peers on adolescent indoor tan-ning behavior: findings from a multi-city sample. J Am Acad Dermatol 2007;57(6):990–7.

50. Cafri G, Thompson JK, Roehrig M, et al. An investi-gation of appearance motives for tanning: the devel-opment and evaluation of the physical appearance reasons for tanning scale (PARTS) and its relation to sunbathing and indoor tanning intentions. Body Image 2006;3(3):199–209.

51. Melamed ML, Michos ED, Post W, et al. 25-Hydrox-yvitamin D levels and the risk of mortality in the gen-eral population. Arch Intern Med 2008;168(15): 1629–37.

52. Freeman S, Francis S, Lundahl K, et al. UV tanning advertisements in high school newspapers. Arch Dermatol 2006;142(4):460–2.

53. Hester EJ, Heilig LF, D'Ambrosia R, et al. Compli-ance with youth access regulations for indoor UV tanning. Arch Dermatol 2005;141(8):959–62.

54. Warthan MM, Uchida T, Wagner RF Jr. UV light tan-ning as a type of substance-related disorder. Arch Dermatol 2005;141(8):963–6.

55. Zeller S, Lazovich D, Forster J, et al. Do adolescent indoor tanners exhibit dependency? J Am Acad Der-matol 2006;54(4):589–96.

56. McLaughlin JA, Francis SO, Burkhardt DL, et al. Indoor UV tanning youth access laws: update 2007. Arch Dermatol 2007;143(4):529–32.

57. Forster JL, Lazovich D, Hickle A, et al. Compliance with restrictions on sale of indoor tanning sessions to youth in Minnesota and Massachusetts. J Am Acad Dermatol 2006;55(6):962–7.

58. Mayer JA, Hoerster KD, Pichon LC, et al. Enforce-ment of state indoor tanning laws in the United States. Prev Chronic Dis 2008;5(4). Available at: http://www.cdc.gov/pcd/issues/2008/oct/07_0194.htm. Accessed January 30, 2009.

59. Howe W, Reed B, Dellavalle RP. Adding over-the-counter dihydroxyacetone self-tanners to sunscreen regimens to increase ultraviolet A light protection. J Am Acad Dermatol 2008;58(5):894.

60. Faurschou A, Wulf HC. Durability of the sun protection factor provided by dihydroxyacetone. Photodermatol Photoimmunol Photomed 2004; 20(5):239–42.

61. Brooks K, Brooks D, Dajani Z, et al. Use of artificial tanning products among young adults. J Am Acad Dermatol 2006;54(6):1060–6.

62. Jung K, Seifert M, Herrling T, et al. UV-generated free radicals (FR) in skin: their prevention by sunscreens and their induction by self-tanning agents. Spectrochim Acta A Mol Biomol Spectrosc 2008; 69(5):1423–8.

63. Stryker JE, Yaroch AL, Moser RP, et al. Prevalence of sunless tanning product use and related behaviors among adults in the United States: results from a national survey. J Am Acad Dermatol 2007;56(3): 387–90.

64. Barsh G, Attardi LD. A healthy tan? N Engl J Med 2007;356(21):2208–10.

65. Gillbro JM, Marles LK, Hibberts NA, et al. Autocrine catecholamine biosynthesis and the beta-adrenoceptor signal promote pigmentation in human epidermal melanocytes. J Invest Dermatol 2004; 123(2):346–53.

66. Wickelgren I. Skin biology: a healthy tan? Science 2007;315(5816):1214–6.

67. Arad S, Konnikov N, Goukassian DA, et al. T-oligos augment UV-induced protective responses in human skin. FASEB J 2006;20(11):1895–7.

68. Green A, Williams G, NËale R, et al. Daily sunscreen application and betacarotene supplementation in prevention of basal-cell and squamous-cell carcinomas of the skin: a randomised controlled trial. Lancet 1999;354(9180):723–9.

69. Garland CF, Garland FC, Gorham ED. Could sunscreens increase melanoma risk? Am J Public Health 1992;82(4):614–5.

Prevention of Nickel Allergy: The Case for Regulation?

Linh K. Lu, MD, PhD[a], Erin M. Warshaw, MD, MS[b],
Cory A. Dunnick, MD[c],*

KEYWORDS

- Metal • Prevalence • Risk factors • Clinical
- Diagnosis • Treatment • Barriers

Nickel is a ubiquitous metal found in the Earth's core as well as in soil, water, and air. It was first discovered in 1751 by Swedish chemist Baron Axel Fredrik Cronstedt.[1] Nickel is used worldwide, mainly in the manufacture of steel, because of its strength and resistance to oxidation. Stainless steel is composed of iron alloyed with at least 10% chromium; other metals such as nickel and molybdenum are often added to prevent staining, rusting, and corrosion. Not only can nickel be combined with stainless steel, but it can also be combined with other transitional metals including cobalt, palladium, iron, titanium, vanadium, and magnesium. Nickel-containing metal alloys are abundant in most industrialized countries and can be found in everyday items such as jewelry, eyeglass frames, watchbands, belt buckles, snaps, and coins. Nickel allergy is the most common metal allergy and the most common overall allergen detected in patch-test populations.[2,3]

PREVALENCE OF NICKEL ALLERGY

The North American Contact Dermatitis Group (NACDG), a group of 13 dermatologists in the United States and Canada, collects de-identified data on patch-tested patients and publishes the epidemiologic data every 2 years. Since 1992, nickel has been the most frequent positive allergen in the group's screening panel of 65 allergens.[2]

Supporting data show that rates of nickel sensitivity have increased over the past decade. In 1992–1995, 14.5% of patients tested had a positive patch test to nickel compared with 18.8% of patients in 2003–2004 ($P<.0001$, **Fig. 1**).[4] Patients under age 18 had significantly higher rates of nickel sensitivity compared with older patients, and women also had significantly higher rates of nickel allergy than men.[4]

Nickel contact dermatitis is common in other industrialized countries. The European Surveillance System on Contact Allergies (ESSCA), a group of dermatologists who collect data on patch-tested patients from nine countries in Europe, reported that nickel sulfate was the most frequently positive allergen and affected 17.3% of patients tested in the years 2002–2003.[3] Within the ESSCA, the highest rates of nickel allergy occurred in Italy (31.7%), where children are exposed to costume jewelry at a young age and where a nickel directive was only implemented in July 2001.[3] The lowest rates of nickel sensitivity were in Denmark (8.1%), probably due to the fact the nickel has been regulated in consumer goods since 1992.[3,5]

IMMUNOLOGY AND GENETICS OF NICKEL ALLERGIC CONTACT DERMATITIS

Allergic contact dermatitis is a type IV reaction, also known as delayed type hypersensitivity. This

There was no grant support for this project and the authors have no conflicts of interest to disclose.
[a] Southern California Permanente Medical Group, 9961 Sierra Avenue, Fontana, CA 92336, USA
[b] University of Minnesota, Department 111K, 1 Veterans Drive, Minneapolis, MN 55417-2309, USA
[c] Department of Dermatology, University of Colorado Denver, 1665 N. Ursula Street, Room 3004, P.O. Box 6510, F703, Aurora, CO 80045, USA
* Corresponding author.
E-mail address: cory.dunnick@ucdenver.edu (C. A. Dunnick).

Dermatol Clin 27 (2009) 155–161
doi:10.1016/j.det.2008.11.003

derm.theclinics.com

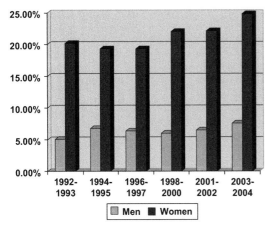

Fig. 1. Rising prevalence of positive patch tests to nickel by gender, NACDG patients. (*Data from* Rietschel RL, Fowler JF, Warshaw EM, et al. Detection of nickel sensitivity has increased in North American patch-test patients. Dermatitis 2008;19:16–9.)

reaction results from skin contact with the metal ions, which bind to proteins of the skin and induce a cellular immune response. Nickel has been shown to elicit a mixed Th1- and Th2-type cytokine response in peripheral blood mononuclear cells (PBMC) from patients with known sensitivity to nickel. In vitro measurements of these responses to nickel have shown increases in expression of IL-2, IL-4, IL-13, and INF-γ from PBMC of sensitized patients.[6] The immunologic response to nickel is similar to that in patients allergic to other metals.[6,7]

Nickel ions act like a conventional peptide in terms of T-cell receptor activation. After nickel has come into contact with the skin, it forms an antigenic complex with a self-peptide and a specific major histocompatibility complex (MHC) molecule on Langerhans cells, which are specialized antigen-presenting cells on the skin. These Langerhans cells then migrate to the draining lymph nodes to sensitize naïve T cells.[8] This specific nickel and MHC–peptide complex is then presented to a repertoire of T-cell receptors, eventually resulting in an inflammatory cascade. A nickel atom is at the center of the complex, forming coordinate bonds with the MHC-peptide complex and the T-cell receptor.[9] Because the activation of the immune response requires specific peptides and MHC molecules, only sensitized individuals develop an allergic reaction to nickel. However, nickel can also activate T cells through other mechanisms that are not dependent on MHC molecules.

Genetic studies of nickel allergy have been inconclusive.[10,11] Some animal research has shown an inherited predisposition to the development of allergic contact dermatitis. Family studies have also shown a tendency toward higher rates of allergic contact dermatitis within related individuals, but such studies have not been able to conclusively control for environmental exposures.[11] In a large female twin study, there was a trend toward concordance for nickel allergy among female monozygotic twins compared with dizygotic twins, but the results were not statistically significant and may have been skewed by the fact that only twins with hand eczema were studied.[12,13] Most experts believe that nickel allergic contact dermatitis is related to environmental exposure rather than genetic factors.[12]

RISK FACTORS FOR CONTACT ALLERGY TO NICKEL

The most important risk factors for developing nickel sensitivity are female sex and younger age. The relative risk is 3.74 in women compared with men (95% CI 3.51–3.98) and the relative risk for those 30 years or less is 3.23 (95% CI 3.03–3.45).[14] However, 12.9% of children under age five (54% boys and 45% girls) were found to be nickel sensitive in a population-based study of 85 children in Denver.[15] This suggests that exposure in childhood does not have the same female predominance as in adult populations. Ear piercing is also an important risk factor for nickel sensitization.[16] A study of 567 Danish citizens found that nickel sensitization was higher among patients with pierced ears (14.8%) compared with those without ear piercings (1.8%).[17] The higher rates of ear piercings in women compared with men is often used to explain the differences in nickel allergy between the sexes. As the popularity of body piercings increases in both sexes, the rate of nickel allergy will also likely increase.

Occupations shown to be at high risk for nickel exposure and sensitization include metal workers, retail clerks, hairdressers, domestic cleaners, and caterers. Tasks performed by metal workers include welding, nickel electroplating, operating machines with metal wires and alloys, engineering metal alloys, lining steel furnaces, metal cutting, and pattern making with metal sheets. Hairdressers handle nickel-plated scissors and other tools. Retail clerks handle metal coins and jewelry. Domestic cleaners and caterers also handle metal objects in the work environment.[18]

CLINICAL PRESENTATION

The most common presentation of nickel contact dermatitis is a well-demarcated, erythematous, papular eczematous plaque at the site of nickel contact. Common locations include the face from eyeglasses, earlobes from earrings, wrist from watches, neck from necklaces, and periumbilical skin from belt buckles, buttons, or snaps (**Figs. 2** and **3**). In the acute state, blisters and weeping may be present, whereas lichenification is typical of chronic exposure. Because Langerhans and T cells circulate throughout the body, areas that are not in direct contact with the allergen can also be affected. This immune-mediated reaction is referred to as autoeczematization or an id reaction (**Fig. 4**). In a small study of 30 children, id reactions were seen in 50% of children with nickel allergic contact dermatitis.[19] The study also found that children as young as age 1 can be sensitized to nickel and that a periumbilical skin eruption was the most common location for the skin rash.

Hand dermatitis due to contact with nickel-plated items such as scissors or coins is not uncommon. Vesicular hand dermatitis due to oral ingestion of nickel in food has also been described but is controversial.[1] Systemic contact dermatitis has also been described with oral ingestion of dietary nickel; the most sensitive patients may react to just 0.22–0.35 mg of daily nickel intake.[20] Foods high in nickel content include whole wheat, oatmeal, chocolate, beans, nuts, and dried fruit. Vitamins may even contain added nickel. Nickel can also leach from cans and stainless steel cooking utensils into foods. The nickel content of fruits and vegetables varies according to soil nickel content. Some authorities recommend a low nickel diet for patients with known nickel allergy.[1]

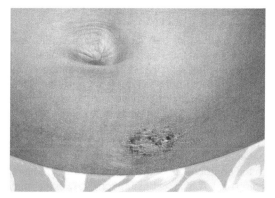

Fig. 3. A classic example of nickel allergic contact dermatitis in the periumbilical area. (*Courtesy of* C. A. Dunnick, MD, Denver, CO.)

NICKEL ALLERGY FROM IMPLANTED METAL DEVICES

Despite the fact that stainless steel is generally considered safe for nickel-sensitive patients, nickel can be released by stainless steel alloys used in medical devices in quantities sufficient to elicit allergic reactions.[21] Furthermore, repeated contact with sweat and saliva may accelerate the release of nickel ions from these stainless steel devices. There are rare reports of orthopedic implants which have caused local and generalized eczematous reactions which have resolved with removal of the metal implant.[22,23] There are also reports of metal-on-metal joint prosthesis failures attributed to nickel allergy, although definitive tests are lacking.[24] Patients may react to dental prostheses as well as orthodontic wires and braces.[21,25] Skin staples and peripheral intravenous catheters may also cause reactions.[26,27] Most concerning is the possibility of metal allergy

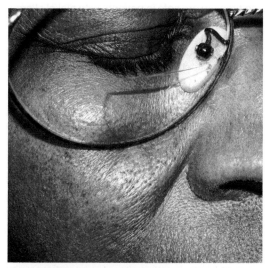

Fig. 2. Allergic contact dermatitis from nickel-containing eyeglass frames. (*Courtesy of* C. A. Dunnick, MD, Denver, CO.)

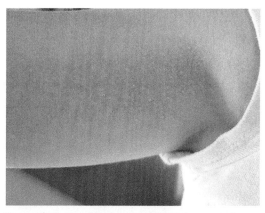

Fig. 4. The same patient as in **Fig. 3** demonstrates an autoeczematization (id) reaction. Note the uniform appearance of the flat-topped papules on the upper arm at a site remote from nickel contact. (*Courtesy of* C. A. Dunnick, MD, Denver, CO.)

contributing to in-stent restenosis of endovascular coronary stents.[28,29]

Due to the fact that incidences of implant-related cutaneous allergies are rare, the epidemiology is not well established.[30] Observations about the relationship between implants and dermatitis have been mostly correlative and shown in case study reports. A study by Reed and colleagues[31] showed that patch testing performed after the implants were placed had limited value, because patients did not have positive patch test results to the components of their implants. Patch testing completed before implantation, however, may provide guidance for selecting implant device materials that will not invoke a reaction. Currently it is unknown whether implants play a causal role in cutaneous metal allergies and there are no set criteria for dealing with cutaneous allergies that may be implant-related.

DIAGNOSIS AND TREATMENT

Nickel allergic contact dermatitis should be considered when dermatitis is present in locations of exposure to nickel-containing products. The standard for diagnosis of allergic contact dermatitis is patch testing. Patch testing involves placing nickel sulfate (2.5% or 5%) in petrolatum in direct contact with the skin for 48 hours and then examining the skin for a local reaction 72 to 96 hours later. Positive reactions exhibit erythema, induration, and papules (**Fig. 5**). Strong positive reactions may even result in a localized vesiculobullous reaction.

Skin biopsy is not necessary for the diagnosis of allergic contact dermatitis. Biopsy findings may support a diagnosis of allergic contact dermatitis, but are not specific as similar reaction patterns can also be seen in drug eruptions and

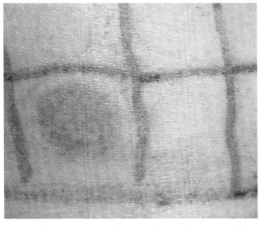

Fig. 5. This patient patch-tested positive to a nickel-containing coin. (*Courtesy of* C. A. Dunnick, MD, Denver, CO.)

eczematous dermatitis. Histology shows spongiosis, mixed dermal inflammatory infiltrate with lymphocytes, histiocytes, and eosinophils, and at times intraepidermal vesiculation and bulla.

The treatment of nickel contact dermatitis is primarily aimed at prevention of the dermatitis through allergen avoidance. However, medical treatment is indicated for symptomatic relief of allergic contact dermatitis. Various studies have shown the effectiveness of potent topical steroids such as fluticasone propionate 0.005% ointment, clobetasol butyrate 0.05% cream, and fluocinonide 0.05% ointment.[32,33] As in the treatment of atopic dermatitis, these topical steroids can be applied twice a day until lesions are resolved, which may take 3 to 4 weeks.[34] Both topical steroids and calcineurin inhibitors have also been shown effective in the treatment of acute areas of allergic contact dermatitis.[35] Antihistamines, such hydroxyzine or cetirizine can be useful to help control pruritus. For a severe acute reaction, such as a vesiculobullus reaction involving more than 10% of the body surface area, systemic steroids may be indicated.[36] Since nickel allergic contact dermatitis is immune mediated with the possibility of new lesions developing for up to 3 weeks, treatment with oral steroids should be tapered over 3 weeks. An allergic flare may result if oral steroids are prematurely discontinued.[37]

PREVENTION

Allergen avoidance is the most effective strategy to avoid nickel contact dermatitis. Elastic can replace metal zippers and buttons in clothing. Generally, stainless steel, sterling silver, platinum, and titanium are safe in patients with nickel allergy. Yellow gold that is less than 18K and white gold may contain allergenic amounts of nickel. Patients should be educated about the availability of a nickel detection kit (dimethylglyoxime [DMG] test). The DMG test is a rapid, easy, and readily available method for detecting nickel in metal objects.[38] DMG on a cotton swab will turn pink if a metal object contains detectable nickel. Patients can test items in the store prior to purchase without harming the item.

Coating a nickel object with a physical barrier may prevent release of nickel ions. Jewelry can be rhodium-plated by a jeweler, but this can wear off over time. Nail polish is commonly recommended as a barrier to coat nickel objects; however, it may be ineffective as it can be washed off, scratched off, or worn away. Recently, four types of barrier coatings (two brands of clear nail polish, super glue, and Nickel Guard) were applied to nickel coins and then assessed for efficacy in yielding negative dimethylglyoxime test results. The investigators found that a nail polish ("Beauty Secrets Hardener") and Nickel Guard were equally effective in yielding a negative DMG test result after applying at least two coats, but Beauty Secrets Hardener was the more cost-effective choice.[39]

If allergen avoidance in clothing is not practical or desirable, an iron-on cloth can be used. Iron-on cloths have been traditionally used to mend holes in clothing and are available in a variety of colors and designs at fabric, arts and crafts, and department stores. As a nickel barrier, it can be ironed on to the inside of the metal portion of clothing. This provides a hidden barrier, unlike sewn-on patches that can show visible stitches on the outside of garments.

Another physical barrier is duct tape. This can adhere to the inside of buttons or snaps. The advantage of duct tape is that it is economical, easy to apply, and widely available. This works well in those articles of clothing that are worn occasionally and require a barrier without much preparation or advanced notice. The disadvantage of duct tape is that the ends may become ragged and cause irritant contact dermatitis with prolonged use. The 11-year-old nickel-allergic patient in **Fig. 6** employed duct tape.

The third technique for preventing nickel allergic contact dermatitis consists of chemical barriers. Barrier creams act either by chelating the positive ionic charge and rendering the metal inactive or by preventing the penetration of nickel through the skin. Nickel chelators have been investigated for their ability to bind nickel and prevent the symptoms of nickel allergic contact dermatitis since 1951.[40] In two reports, pretreatment with disodium ethylenediamine tetra-acetate blocked the effect of nickel-induced allergic contact dermatitis

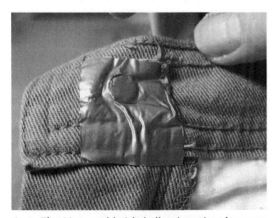

Fig. 6. The 11-year-old nickel-allergic patient here employed duct tape as a physical barrier for the nickel containing button at the waistline of these pants. (*Courtesy of* C. A. Dunnick, MD, Denver, CO.)

during a patch test.[41,42] In another study of 28 nickel sensitized patients, pretreatment with 10% diethylenetriaminepentaacetic acid decreased nickel-specific patch test reaction.[43]

With respect to nonchelating barrier creams, the rationale for their effect is that they provide protection against the invasion of foreign products, such as nickel, and against excessive transepidermal water loss. Application of a moisturizing cream (a non-ionic oil-in-water emulsion containing 9% glycerin and 4% evening primrose oil) after a nickel-mediated patch test reaction resulted in significantly better recovery of the disrupted skin with reduced transepidermal water loss in the 12 patients tested.[44] Regular use of skin moisturizers may also help prevent skin barrier damage in nickel allergic patients.[45] The absorption of nickel through the skin can also be decreased with a cream containing propylene glycol, petrolatum, and lanolin.[46] More studies are necessary to determine efficacy of chelating and nonchelating barrier creams in nickel contact dermatitis.

PRIMARY PREVENTION AND REGULATION OF NICKEL IN CONSUMER ITEMS

Because of the increasing prevalence of nickel sensitivity, several European countries have implemented regulations to limit the amount of nickel released from jewelry and other objects in close contact with the skin. The European Union Nickel Directive was adopted in 1994 and limits the amount to no more than 0.05% nickel content in posts used for body piercings. Furthermore, it limits the amount of nickel released from objects in direct and prolonged contact with the skin to no more than 0.5 μg nickel/cm^2/week. It also mandates that these objects, such as jewelry, watches, buttons, and zippers, shall maintain this requirement for 2 years of normal use.[47]

Regulation of nickel has successfully lowered rates of nickel sensitization. In Germany, nickel allergy in women under age 30 decreased significantly from 36.7% (in 1992) to 25.8% (in 2001).[48] In Denmark, nickel sensitivity in children under age 18 fell from 24.8% to 9.2% from 1985–1986 to 1997–1998.[49] Danish schoolgirls whose ears were pierced prior to nickel regulation in 1992 had an odds ratio of 3.34 for nickel sensitization in contrast to girls whose ears were pierced after regulation (OR 1.2).[5] In the same study, 250 items of jewelry were tested with DMG and none released nickel, indicating successful compliance by jewelry manufacturers. Another study in Sweden documented that in 1999, 25% of 725 items tested positive for released nickel whereas only 8% of 786 items tested positive for nickel in 2002–2003 after nickel regulation was introduced.[50]

To raise awareness about nickel allergy, the American Contact Dermatitis Society named nickel the 2008 Contact Allergen of the Year[51] and has sponsored resolutions recommending limits in consumer products similar to those adopted in Europe. The American Academy of Dermatology is considering this resolution for adoption as part of its platform.

SUMMARY

Nickel is the most common allergen detected in patch-tested patients, affecting up to 35.8% of young females in this group. Management of nickel allergy consists of avoidance and barrier methods. Successful primary prevention will likely require governmental regulation of nickel content in consumer items.

REFERENCES

1. Sharma AD. Relationship between nickel allergy and diet. Indian J Dermatol 2007;73(5):307–12.
2. Pratt MD, Belsito DV, DeLeo VA, et al. North American contact dermatitis group patch test results, 2001–2002 study period. Dermatitis 2004;15(4):176–83.
3. Uter W, Hegewald J, Aberer W, et al. The European standard series in 9 European countries, 2002/2003 – First results of the European surveillance system on contact allergies. Contact Derm 2005;53:136–45.
4. Rietschel RL, Fowler JF, Warshaw EM, et al. Detection of nickel sensitivity has increased in North American patch-test patients. Dermatitis 2008;19(1):16–9.
5. Jensen CS, Lisby S, Baadsgaard O, et al. Decrease in nickel sensitization in a Danish schoolgirl population with ears pierced after implementation of a nickel-exposure regulation. Br J Dermatol 2002; 146:636–42.
6. Minang JT, Arestrom I, Troye-Blomberg M, et al. Nickel, cobalt, chromium, palladium and gold induce a mixed Th1- and Th2-type cytokine response in vitro in subjects with contact allergy to the respective metals. Clin Exp Immunol 2006;146: 417–26.
7. Gawkrodger DJ, Lewis FM, Shah M. Contact hypersensitivity to nickel and other metal in jewelry reactors. J Am Acad Dermatol 2000;43:31–6.
8. Boisleve F, Kerdine-Romer S, Rougier-Larzat N, et al. Nickel and DNCB induce CCR7 expression on human dendritic cells through different signalling pathways: role of TNF-alpha and MAPK. J Invest Dermatol 2004;123:494–502.
9. Lu L, Vollmer J, Moulon C, et al. Components of the ligand of a Ni++ reactive human T cell clone. J Exp Med 2003;197:567–74.
10. Liden S, Beckman L, Cedergren B, et al. Lack of association between allergic contact dermatitis and HLA antigens of the A and B series. Acta Derm Venereol 1981;61:155–7.
11. Schram AE, Warshaw EM. Genetics of nickel allergic contact dermatitis. Dermatitis 2007;18(3):125–33.
12. Bryld LE, Hindsberger C, Kyvik KO, et al. Genetic factors in nickel allergy evaluated in a population-based female twin sample. J Invest Dermatol 2004;123:1025–9.
13. Bataille V. Genetic factors in nickel allergy. J Invest Dermatol 2004;123(6):xxiv–v.
14. Uter W, Pfahlberg A, Gefeller O, et al. Risk factors for contact allergy to nickel – results of a multifactorial analysis. Contact Derm 2003;48:33–8.
15. Bruckner AL, Weston WL, Morelli JG. Does sensitization to contact allergens begin in infancy? Pediatrics 2000;105(1):1–4.
16. Matilla L, Kilpelainen M, Terho EO, et al. Prevalence of nickel allergy among Finnish university students in 1995. Contact Derm 2001;44:218–23.
17. Neilsen NH, Menne T. Nickel sensitisation and ear-piercing in an unselected Danish population. Glostrup allergy study. Contact Derm 1993;29:16–21.
18. Shah M, Lewis FM, Gawkrodger DJ. Nickel as an occupational allergen. Arch Dermatol 1998;134:1231–6.
19. Silverberg NB, Licht J, Friedler S, et al. Nickel contact hypersensitivity in children. Pediatr Dermatol 2002;19(2):110–3.
20. Jensen CS, Menne T, Johansen JD. Systemic contact dermatitis after oral exposure to nickel: a review with a modified meta-analysis. Contact Derm 2006;54:79–86.
21. Jensen CS, Lisby S, Baadsgaard O, et al. Release of nickel ions from stainless steel alloys used in dental braces and their patch test reactivity in nickel-sensitive individuals. Contact Derm 2003;48:300–4.
22. Kanerva L, Forstrom L. Allergic nickel and chromate hand dermatitis induced by orthopaedic metal implant. Contact Derm 2001;44:103–4.
23. Thomas P, Gollwitzer H, Maier S, et al. Osteosynthesis associated with contact dermatitis with unusual perpetuation of hyperreactivity in a nickel allergic patient. Contact Derm 2006;54:222–5.
24. Gawkrodger DJ. Metal sensitivities and orthopaedic implants revisited: the potential for metal allergy with the new metal-on-metal joint prostheses. Br J Dermatol 2003;148:1089–93.
25. Yesudian PD, Memon A. Nickel-induced angular cheilitis due to orthodontic braces. Contact Derm 2003;48(1):287–8.
26. Conde-Salazar L, Valks R, Malfeito JE, et al. Contact dermatitis from the staples of neuroreflexotherapy. Contact Derm 2004;51(4):217–8.
27. Raison-Peyron N, Guillard O, Khalil Z, et al. Nickel-elicited systemic contact dermatitis from a peripheral intravenous catheter. Contact Derm 2005;53:222–5.

28. Ekqvist S, Svedman C, Moller H, et al. High frequency of contact allergy to gold in patients with endovascular coronary stents. Br J Dermatol 2007;157:730–8.

29. Koster A, Schomig A, Dirschinger J, et al. Nickel and molybdenum contact allergies in patients with coronary in-stent restenosis. Lancet 2000;356:1895–7.

30. Thomas P, Schuh A, Ring J, et al. Orthopedic surgical implants and allergies: joint statement by the Implant Allergy Working Group (AK 20) of the DGOOC (German Association of Orthopedics and Orthopedic Surgery), DKG (German Contact Dermatitis Research Group) and DGAKI (German Society for Allergology and Clinical Immunology). Orthopade 2008;37(1):75–88.

31. Reed KB, Davis MD, Nakamura K, et al. Retrospective evaluation of patch testing before or after metal device implantation. Arch Dermatol 2008;144(8):999–1007.

32. Hachem JP, De Paepe K, Vanpee E, et al. Efficacy of topical corticosteroids in nickel-induced contact allergy. Clin Exp Dermatol 2002;27:47–50.

33. Parneix-Spake A, Goustas P, Green R. Eumovate (clobetasone butyrate) 0.05% cream with its moisturizing emollient base has better healing properties than hydrocortisone 1% cream: a study in nickel-induced contact dermatitis. J Dermatolog Treat 2001;12:191–7.

34. Saary J, Qureshi R, Palda V, et al. A systematic review of contact dermatitis treatment and prevention. J Am Acad Dermatol 2005;53:845–55.

35. Bhardwaj SS, Jaimes JP, Liu A, et al. A double-blind randomized placebo-controlled pilot study comparing topical immunomodulating agents and corticosteroids for treatment of experimentally induced nickel contact dermatitis. Dermatitis 2007;18(1):26–31.

36. Bruckner AL, Weston WL. Allergic contact dermatitis in children: a practical approach to management. Skin Therapy Lett 2002;7:3–5.

37. Mowad CM, Marks JG Jr. Allergic contact dermatitis. In: Bolognia JL, Jorizzo JL, Rapini RP, editors. Dermatology. New York: Mosby; 2003. p. 227–40.

38. Allergan's true test patient information templates: nickel sulfate. Available at: http://www.truetest.com/PatientPDF/Patient_Nickel.pdf. Accessed January 15, 2009.

39. Sprigle AM, Marks JG, Anderson BE. Prevention of nickel release with barrier coatings. Dermatitis 2008;19(1):28–31.

40. Rostenberg A Jr, Perkins AJ. Nickel and cobalt dermatitis. J Allergy 1951;22:466–74.

41. van Ketel WG, Bruynzeel DP. Chelating effect of EDTA on nickel. Contact Derm 1984;11:311–4.

42. Fullerton A, Menne T. In vitro and in vivo evaluation of the effect of barrier gels in nickel contact allergy. Contact Derm 1995;32:100–6.

43. Wohrl S, Kriechbaumer N, Hemmer W, et al. A cream containing the chelator DTPA (diethylenetriamine-penta-acetic acid) can prevent contact allergic reactions to metals. Contact Derm 2001;44:224–8.

44. De Paepe K, Hachem JP, Vanpee E, et al. Beneficial effects of a skin tolerance-tested moisturizing cream on the barrier function in experimentally-elicited irritant and allergic contact dermatitis. Contact Derm 2001;44:337–43.

45. Hachem JP, De Paepe K, Vanpee E, et al. The effect of two moisturisers on skin barrier damage in allergic contact dermatitis. Eur J Dermatol 2002;12:136–8.

46. Gawkrodger DJ, Healey J, Howe AM. The prevention of nickel contact dermatitis. A review of the use of binding agents and barrier creams. Contact Derm 1995;32(5):257–65.

47. Liden C. Legislative and preventive measures related to contact dermatitis. Contact Derm 2001;44:65–9.

48. Schnuch A, Uter W. Decrease in nickel allergy in Germany and regulatory interventions. Contact Derm 2003;49(2):107–8.

49. Johansen JD, Menne T, Christophersen J, et al. Changes in the pattern of sensitization to common contact allergens in Denmark between 1985–86 and 1997–98, with a special view to preventive strategies. Br J Dermatol 2000;142:490–5.

50. Liden C, Norberg K. Nickel on the Swedish market. Follow up after implementation of the nickel directive. Dermatitis 2005;52:29–35.

51. Kronik R, Zug KA. Nickel. Dermatitis 2008;19(1):3–8.

Teledermatology: A Review of Reliability and Accuracy of Diagnosis and Management

Yakir S. Levin, PhD[a], Erin M. Warshaw, MD, MS[b],*

KEYWORDS

- Teledermatology • Accuracy • Health services research
- Telemedicine • Reliability

Telemedicine, broadly defined, uses telecommunication technology to transfer medical information. Multiple fields, including ophthalmology, radiology, pathology, psychiatry, and dermatology, use telemedicine to enable medical diagnosis or treatment by a physician located at some distance from the patient. Several motivations guide the use of telecommunication in dermatology, also known as teledermatology. First, it provides geographically isolated patients access to dermatology. Urban areas in the United States[1] and in Canada[2] enjoy a relative abundance of dermatologists compared with rural areas. Teledermatology could help rectify this imbalance in access. Second, primary care settings may use teledermatology to triage cases and limit unnecessary referrals to dermatologists. Long wait times for appointments with dermatologists exist in rural and urban areas,[3] and eliminating unnecessary referrals may ease demand. Third, teledermatology could provide an avenue for direct follow-up care at a distance (eg, leg ulcer monitoring).

The use of teledermatology dates back to 1972, when university-based dermatologists saw employees at Boston's Logan Airport by way of a live black-and-white video link.[4] During the 1980s, advances such as analog-to-digital conversion, which allowed compression of video and still images, and increasing transmission bandwidth made teledermatology a practical consideration. Between 1993 and 1998, the Association of Telemedicine Service Providers documented a total of at least 44 teledermatology programs in 30 states, a 15-fold increase in the number of active telemedicine programs in the United States. In 1998, at least 58,000 telemedicine interactions occurred in the United States, including 3316 teledermatology encounters.[5] Despite this increase, these consultations represented only 0.00042% of all ambulatory care visits and only slightly more than a month's work for one busy general dermatologist.[6] In 2003, 36 states (70%) had a total of 58 teledermatology programs, most of which were affiliated with academic centers.[7]

Modern teledermatology uses two different modalities: live interactive teledermatology and store-and-forward teledermatology. Live interactive teledermatology uses video-conferencing equipment to connect patient and dermatologist in real time. Store-and-forward teledermatology uses still images sent to a dermatologist, who reviews them and provides recommendations at a later time. Table 1 compares the two modalities.

The purpose of this article is to summarize the published literature on the reliability and accuracy of teledermatology. Although we did not do a formal

The views expressed in this article are those of the authors and do not necessarily reflect the position or policy of the Department of Veterans Affairs.

a Stanford University Schools of Medicine and Engineering, Palo Alto, CA 94305, USA

b Department of Dermatology, Minneapolis Veterans Affairs Medical Center, 111K, One Veterans Drive, Minneapolis, MN 55417, USA

* Corresponding author.

E-mail address: erin.warshaw@med.va.gov (E.M. Warshaw).

Dermatol Clin 27 (2009) 163–176

doi:10.1016/j.det.2008.11.012

0733-8635/08/$ – see front matter. Published by Elsevier Inc.

derm.theclinics.com

Table 1
Comparison of live interactive and store-and-forward teledermatology systems

	Live Interactive	Store and Forward
Camera	Video camera	Digital still camera
Images	Live, streaming video	Still photographs
Teledermatologist interaction with patient	Live, by way of video link	None, written comments sent to referring provider
Relative cost	Expensive	Inexpensive
Coordination	Imager, patient, and teledermatologist must all be available at the same time	Teledermatologist may review history and images at his/her convenience
Federal Medicare reimbursement	Yes	No (except in Hawaii and Alaska); used primarily in military and veterans affairs medical care systems

systematic review, we conducted a literature search using the terms "teledermatology" and "telemedicine and dermatology" in PubMed in the spring of 2008. Full texts of all articles published in English were retrieved and reviewed by both authors. We limited this review to those studies that compared diagnosis or management; they excluded publications focused on technology, implementation, satisfaction,[8–17] or economic outcomes (unless agreement or accuracy were used as outcomes of effectiveness).[18–28] Readers interested in camera specifications and guidelines will find a wealth of information on the World Wide Web.[29,30]

The article is divided into four sections. The first section reports on the diagnostic reliability of teledermatology compared with face-to-face clinic consultation. Diagnostic reliability refers specifically to diagnostic reproducibility, or diagnostic agreement, between dermatologists using the two different modalities. The authors defined matching of the primary diagnosis of the clinic dermatologist and the primary diagnosis of the teledermatologist as "complete agreement." They defined "partial agreement" as matching of any of the clinic dermatologist's diagnoses (primary or differential diagnoses) with any of the teledermatologist's diagnoses (primary or differential diagnosis). The second section reports on the "intragroup" diagnostic agreement between either clinic dermatologists or teledermatologists and serves as a basis for comparison of the results of the first section. The third section reports on the diagnostic accuracy for those studies that include definitive histopathologic diagnosis. The last section summarizes the literature comparing clinical management decisions by clinic dermatologists to those made by teledermatologists.

DIAGNOSTIC AGREEMENT RATES BETWEEN TELEDERMATOLOGISTS AND CLINIC-BASED DERMATOLOGISTS

For teledermatology to gain acceptance in situations where it is applied in lieu of in-person dermatologic care, it should ideally perform as well as clinic-based dermatology. Studies on diagnostic agreement compare diagnoses of teledermatologists with clinic-based dermatologists. Investigators report their results as simple percent agreement or with kappa (κ) statistics ($\kappa \leq 0.2$ poor; 0.21–0.40 fair; 0.41–0.60 moderate; 0.61–0.80 good; 0.81–01.00 very good agreement).[31] **Table 2**[32–67] summarizes these results. Comparisons of studies are complicated by several variables, including the teledermatologic system (store and forward or live interactive); the number and level of training of clinic dermatologists and teledermatologists; and the method of assessing diagnostic agreement. In several studies, the same dermatologist served as both clinic dermatologist and teledermatologist, either exclusively,[33,50,52,55,60] or in only some cases.[32,35,61,68] In these instances, agreement between clinic dermatologist and teledermatologist represents "intraobserver" agreement and thus controls for different diagnostic tendencies among different dermatologists. However, these cases necessarily involve bias because the clinic dermatologist has usually seen the digital images before seeing the patient. Studies also differed in the inclusion of teledermatoscopy[44,56–58,69] and in the types of skin conditions (eg, multiple dermatologic conditions including rashes, pigmented lesions only,[56,57,69,70] or neoplasms in general).[36,44,47,54,58,67,71] Overall, teledermatologists and clinic dermatologists completely agreed with each other in 41%[38] to 94%[57] of cases. They had partial agreement in 50%[35] to 100%.[53]

When two groups of clinic dermatologists (eight different residents and four different staff) and three staff teledermatologists examined 129 patients who had 168 skin conditions using store-and-forward teledermatology, complete diagnostic agreement ranged from 41% to 55% and partial agreement ranged from 79% to 95%.[38] In another store-and-forward study of 121 skin conditions in 116 patients, 1 of 13 clinic dermatologists and one of two teledermatologists evaluated each patient. The two teledermatologists completely agreed with the clinic dermatologist in 61% and 64% of cases, respectively, whereas they partially agreed in 67% and 70%.[40] Higher confidence level correlated well with better agreement rates. In a study of live interactive teledermatology that evaluated 351 patients who had 427 skin conditions, clinic dermatologists and teledermatologists completely agreed in 67% and partially agreed in 82% of cases.[59] In another study of live interactive teledermatology, involving 135 skin conditions in 104 patients, the same person served as teledermatologist and clinic dermatologist in 79% of cases. Overall, the teledermatologist completely agreed with the clinic dermatologist in 75% of cases and partially agreed in 82% of cases.[63] One melanoma (subsequently biopsy proved) was missed by teledermatology and 11 of the 16 (69%) incorrect diagnoses were benign and malignant skin neoplasms.

INTRAGROUP DIAGNOSTIC AGREEMENT RATES BETWEEN CLINIC DERMATOLOGISTS OR BETWEEN TELEDERMATOLOGISTS

Teledermatology should not be evaluated solely on agreement between teledermatologists and clinic-based dermatologists.[15] Because examiners disagree with each other to some extent in any consult modality, we must place the level of agreement between teledermatologists and clinic-based examiners in the context of agreement among clinic-based examiners. **Table 3** (see Refs.[32,34,38,39,44,52–55,57,65,72]) lists studies reporting interobserver agreement between clinic dermatologists and between teledermatologists (intragroup agreement). Among all studies, clinic dermatologists completely agreed with each other in 54% to 95% of cases and partially agreed with each other in 90% to 100%. Teledermatologists demonstrated complete agreement in 46%[53] to 83%,[57] and partial agreement in 84%[38] to 92%.[53] Five studies reported agreement among teledermatologists using κ values; these ranged

from 0.22[39] to 0.91.[55] Note that computation of the κ statistic requires categoric information (eg, benign versus malignant) and does not allow for differential diagnoses. As a result, the reported κ statistics necessarily involved complete agreement.

Several studies reported intragroup agreement among clinic dermatologists. In one study of 72 patients,[44] the investigators reported diagnostic agreement between two clinic dermatologists of 79%, significantly better than the 55% agreement between clinic dermatologists and teledermatologists for a separate group of 92 patients ($P = .002$). A second study similarly compared agreement between clinic dermatologists with agreement between clinic-based and teledermatologists using two separate groups of patients.[65] However, this study differed from the prior one in that the same two dermatologists functioned as clinic dermatologists and teledermatologists. Each clinician served as the teledermatologist for half of the patients and as the clinic dermatologist for the other half of the study. The investigators concluded that intragroup diagnostic agreement for clinic dermatologists (94%) exceeded the diagnostic agreement between teledermatologists and clinic dermatologists (78%) when considering only complete agreement. However, the two groups performed comparably well when including partial agreement in the analysis (100% intragroup agreement between clinic dermatologists, and 99% between teledermatologist and clinic dermatologist). One study of store-and-forward teledermatology[15] found intragroup complete or partial agreement of 84% to 92% among three teledermatologists, and of 92% for two clinic dermatologists, which compared favorably to agreement between clinic dermatologists and teledermatologists of 79% to 95% in the same study.

DIAGNOSTIC ACCURACY

Table 4 (see Refs.[33,34,38,48,53,55,56,58,64,69,72–78]) lists data from studies of teledermatology with reported accuracy rates based on a gold standard (primarily histopathology). These data are especially important for neoplasms, for which histology is the accepted gold standard and where misdiagnosis can lead to significant morbidity and potential mortality. Accuracy rates ranged from 30%[73] to 92%[56] for clinic dermatologists and from 19%[33] to 95% for teledermatologists.[72] In one study evaluating teledermatoscopy of 157 pigmented lesions including 32 melanomas, three teledermatologists with varying levels of dermatoscopy training viewed dermatoscopic images of each lesion.[77] The most experienced had the

Table 2
Diagnostic agreement rates of teledermatologists and clinic dermatologists

Study	No. of Patients	No. of Dermatologic Conditions	No. of Clinic Dermatologists Compared[a]	No. of Teledermatologists Compared[a]	Comparison	Percent Agreement[b] Complete	Partial
Store-and-forward studies							
Baba[32]	228	242 (47 neoplasms)	1 (same as T_1)	2	C_1T_1	81%	NR
					C_1T_2	75%	NR
Pak[33]	404	404 (169 neoplasms)	1 (same as T)	1 (same as C)	C_1T_1	70%	91%
					C_1T_1[c]	76%	92%
Krupinski[34]	308	308	1 (3)	3	C_1T_1	NR	84%
					C_1T_2	NR	85%
					C_1T_3	NR	81%
Baba[32] SF + LI	228	242 (47 neoplasms)	1 (same as T_1)	2	C_1T_1	90%	NR
					C_1T_2	82%	NR
Taylor[35]	183	188	1 (2)	2 (1 same as C)	C_1T_1	31%	50%
					C_1T_2	44%	57%
					C_2T_1	51%	61%
					C_2T_2	64%	70%
					$C_{1,2}T_{1,2}$	51%	63%
Mahendran[36]	163	163 (neoplasms)	1 (2)	2 (3) (T_2 = resident)	C_1T_1	48%	65%
					C_1T_2	44%	64%
Harrison[37]	137	NR	—	—		Overall 84%	
Whited[38]	129	168	2 (C_1 = 1 of 8 residents; C_2 = 1 of 4 staff)	3	C_1T_1	44%	83%
					C_1T_2	46%	79%
					C_1T_3	55%	92%
					C_2T_1	41%	84%
					C_2T_2	44%	83%
					C_2T_3	52%	95%
Oztas[39]	125	125 (18 neoplasms)	1	3	C_1T_1	69%	NR
					C_1T_2	62%	NR
					C_1T_3	80%	NR
Kvedar[40]	116	121	1 (13)	2	C_1T_1	64%	70%
					C_1T_2	61%	67%

Study	N	Lesions/Description	Teledermatologist	Comparator	Comparison	Agreement	Agreement
Du Moulin[41]	106	NR	1 (8)	1	C_1T_1	54%	63%
Lyon[42]	100	100 (38 rashes 62 neoplasms)	1 (resident)	1	C_1T_1 Rash C_1T_1 Neoplasm	NR NR	90% 96%
High[43]	92	106	1 (>1)	3	C_1T_1 C_1T_2 C_1T_3	70% 64% 77%	82% 73% 89%
Bowns[44]	92	NR	1 (>1)	NR		Overall 55%	
Tucker[45]	75	84	1 (2)	1 (2)	C_1T_1	56%	68%
Chao[46]	NR	71	10 ("junior doctors")	5		Overall 95%	
Lewis[47]	56	NR(neoplasms)	NR	NR	C_1T_1	93%ᵈ	
Barnard[48]	50	NR	1 (3)	8	C_1T_{1-8}	77% (67–84)	90% (84–96)
Rashid[49]	33	33 (4 neoplasms)	1 (NR)	1 (NR)	C_1T_1	82%	88%
Tait[50]	NR	30	1 (3) (same as T)	1 (3) (same as C)	C_1T_1	83%	100%
Zelickson[51]	29	30 (18 rashes, 12 neoplasms)	1	2 or 3	C_1T_{1-3}	NR	88%
Lim[52]	25	27	1 (same as T)	1 (same as C)		Overall 88%	
Whited[53]	12	13 (suspected skin cancers)	2	2	C_1T_1 C_1T_2 C_2T_1 C_2T_2	80% 60% 77% 39%	90% 100% 100% 100%
Moreno-Ramirez[54]	882	NR (neoplasms)	1	1	κ = 0.81 (0.78, 0.84)		
Moreno-Ramirez[55]	108	108 (pigmented lesions)	1 (same as T)	1 (same as C)	κ = 0.93 (0.87, 0.96)		
Store-and-forward teledermatoscopy studies							
Bowns[44]	256	256 (suspected skin cancers)	1 (7)	1 (3)	C_1T_1	69%	NR
Piccolo[56]	NR	66 (pigmented lesions)	1 (consensus of 2)	1	C_1T_1	90%	NR
Massone[57]	18	18 (pigmented lesions, 2 MM)	1	2	C_1T_1 C_1T_2	89% 94%	NR NR
Fabbrocini[58]	NR	44 (difficult pink lesions)	2	2	SF: κ = 0.36 (CI: NR) TDMS: κ = 0.44 (CI: NR)		

(continued on next page)

Table 2 (*continued*)

Study	No. of Patients	No. of Dermatologic Conditions	No. of Clinic Dermatologists Compared[a]	No. of Teledermatologists Compared[a]	Percent Agreement[b]		
					Comparison	Complete	Partial
Live interactive studies							
Loane[59]	351	427	1 (>1) (some same as T)	1 (>1) (some same as C)	C_1T_1	67%	82%
Loane[60]	130	153 (32 neoplasms)	1 (same as T)	1 (same as C)	C_1T_1	67%	82%
Gilmour[61]	126	155	1 (5) (some same as T)	1 (NR) (some same as C)	C_1T_1	57%	78%
Nordal[62]	112	112	1	1	C_1T_1	72%	87%
Oakely[63]	104	135	1	2 (79% same as C)	C_1T_1	75%	82%
Lowitt[64]	102	130	1 (2 residents, 2 staff)	1 (2 residents, 2 staff)	C_1T_1	NR	80%
Lesher[65]	60	68	1 (2)	1 (2)	C_1T_1	78%	99%
Phillips[66]	60	79	1 (NR)	1 (2)	C_1T_1 C_1T_2	81% 75%	NR NR
Phillips[67]	51	107 (skin neoplasms)	2	2	Complete: 59% $\kappa = 0.32$ (CI: NR)		

Abbreviations: C, clinic dermatologist; LI, live interactive; MM, malignant melanoma; NR, not reported; SF, store and forward; T, teledermatologist; TDMS, teledermatoscopy.
[a] Number in parentheses represents the total number of dermatologists involved.
[b] Simple percent agreement except for those studies reporting κ statistics (95% CI).
[c] Considering neoplasms alone.
[d] Agreement for benign or malignant status on 1 to 5 rating scale.

Table 3
Intragroup agreement between clinic dermatologists or between teledermatologists

Study	No. of Patients	No. of Skin Conditions	Clinic Dermatologists[a] % Agreement			Teledermatologists[a] % Agreement		
			—	Complete	Partial	—	Complete	Partial
Store-and-forward studies								
Baba[32]	228	242 (47 neoplasms)	NR			SF $\kappa_{12} = 0.71$ (0.60–0.82) SF + LI $\kappa_{12} = 0.79$ (0.70–0.88)		
Krupinski[34]	308	308	NR			$\kappa_{12} = 0.82$, $\kappa_{23} = 0.80$, $\kappa_{13} = 0.81$		
Whited[38]	129	168	— C_1C_2	54%	92%	T_1T_2 T_1T_3 T_2T_3	49% 55% 54%	84% 92% 87%
Oztas[39]	125	125 (18 neoplasms)	NR			T_1T_2 T_1T_3 T_2T_3 $\kappa_{12} = 0.25$, $\kappa_{13} = 0.32$, $\kappa_{23} = 0.22$	55% 70% 67%	NR NR NR
Bowns[44]	72	NR	C_1C_2	79%	NR	NR		
Lim[52]	49	53	NR			T_1T_{2-5}	79%	86%
Whited[53]	12	13 (neoplasms)	C_1C_2	80%	90%	T_1T_2	46%	92%
Moreno-Ramirez[54]	340	340 (neoplasms)	NR			$\kappa_{12} = 0.85$ (0.79–0.91)		
Moreno-Ramirez[55]	219	219 (pigmented neoplasms)	NR			$\kappa = 0.91$ (0.87–0.96)		
Store-and-forward teledermatoscopy studies								
Massone[57]	18	18 (pigmented neoplasms, 2 MM)	NR			T_1T_2	83%	NR
Piccolo[72]	NR	20 (acral pigmented neoplasms)	NR			κ range: 0.49–0.88		
Live interactive studies								
Lesher[65]	36	47	C_1C_2	94%	100%	NR		

Abbreviations: C, clinic dermatologist; LI, live interactive; MM, malignant melanoma; NR, not reported; SF, store and forward; T, teledermatologist.
[a] Number of clinic dermatologists and teledermatologists are listed in Table 2, except for Shapiro, which included 2 teledermatologists, and Piccolo, which involved agreement among 16 teledermatologists.

Table 4
Teledermatology studies reporting accuracy rates involving a gold standard of histopathology

| Study | No. of Patients | No. of Lesions | | Clinic Dermatologist Diagnostic Accuracy Rate | | | Teledermatologist Diagnostic Accuracy Rate | |
				Complete	Partial		Complete	Partial
Store-and-forward studies								
Krupinski[34]	104	NR	C_{1-3}	89%	NR	T_{1-3}	76%	NR
			C_1	80%	NR	T_1	78%	NR
			C_2	97%	NR	T_2	76%	NR
			C_3	90%	NR	T_3	73%	NR
Whited[38]	NR	79 (66 biopsied)	C_1	71%	85%	T_1	53%	68%
			C_2	59%	85%	T_2	63%	78%
						T_3	62%	85%
Barnard[48]	25	25 (8 skin cancers)	C	84%	NR	T	73%	NR
Whited[53]	12	13	C_1	70%	80%	T_1	31%	85%
			C_2	57%	92%	T_2	85%	85%
Moreno-Ramirez[55]	57	57	—	NR			$\kappa = 0.79\ (0.70–0.89)$	
Piccolo[69]	40	43 (pigmented lesions, 11 MM)	C	91%	NR	T_1	88%	NR
			MM: 73%			T_2	95%	NR
						MM: T_1:73%, T_2:81%		
Lozzi[73]	33	33 difficult cases (8 neoplasms)	C_1	42%	NR	T_{1-4}	79%	NR
			C_2	30%	NR	T not blinded to C diagnosis		
Bauer[74]	311	315 (42 MM)	Malignant vs. benign MM: 79% Benign: 96%			NR		

			C same as T C_1			C same as T T_1		
Jolliffe[75]	138	144 (pigmented lesions)	C_1	43%	NR	T_1	47%	NR
Store-and-forward teledermatoscopy studies								
Piccolo[56]	NR	66 (pigmented lesions)	C	92%	NR	T	86%	NR
Fabbrocini[58]	NR	44 (difficult "pink" lesions)	Complete SF κ = 0.52 (CI: NR) Complete TDMS κ = 0.70 (CI: NR) 66% "correct diagnosis"	NR		SF κ = 0.44 (CI: NR) TDMS κ = 0.45 (CI: NR) 52% "correct diagnosis"	86%	NR
Piccolo[69]	40	43 (pigmented lesions)	C MM: 73% κ = 0.74	91%	NR	T_{1-11} κ range = 0.35–0.87	77%–95%	NR
Piccolo[72]	71	77 (melanocytic acral nevi)		NR		T	95%	NR
Piccolo[76]	NR	20	C	85%	NR	T	78%	NR
Blum[77]	NR	157 (pigmented lesions, 32 MM)	NR			T_1 T_2 T_3 MM: T_1:84%, T_2:88%, T_3:84%	90% 89% 87%	NR NR NR
Braun[78]	51	55 (pigmented lesions)	C_{1-6}	64%	NR	T_1	75%	NR
Live interactive studies								
Lowitt[64]	NR	11	C_1	64%	NR	T_1	73%	NR

Abbreviations: C, clinic dermatologist; MM, malignant melanoma; NR, not reported; SF, store and forward; T, teledermatologist; TDMS, teledermatoscopy.

best accuracy (90% versus 89% and 87%) overall, and accuracy rates for melanoma were similar (84% versus 88% versus 84%). A second study[56] evaluated teledermatoscopy of 66 pigmented lesions, which were subsequently examined histo-pathologically. Clinic dermatology accuracy was 92% compared with teledermatology accuracy of 86%. The clinic dermatologists missed two mela-nomas, whereas the teledermatologists did not miss any. A third study[78] compared six clinic dermatologists who had some dermatoscopic experience with an expert teledermatoscopist in their evaluation of 55 pigmented lesions. Diag-nostic accuracy of the expert teledermatoscopist exceeded that of the less experienced participants (75% versus 64%).

MANAGEMENT PLAN AGREEMENT RATES

Appropriateness of clinical management may be the most important criterion by which teledermatology should be evaluated. For example, the decision as to whether to biopsy a lesion may have a greater impact on clinical outcome than accuracy of the clinical diagnosis. Complete 100% agreement in management plans among clinic dermatologists (intragroup agreement) was reported in a study of 12 patients.[53] In a larger study,[38] the investigators divided clinical management plans into three categories: diagnostic testing recommendations, recommendations for medical therapy, and recommendations for clinic-based therapy. Reported agreement in diagnostic testing recommendations among clinic dermatologists was 85%. Recommendations for medical therapy and clinic-based therapy were in agreement for 85% and 77% of clinic dermatologists, respectively.

Four studies reported on agreement in management plans among teledermatologists. Whited and colleagues[38] found agreement among three tele-dermatologist pairs of 73% to 75%, 64% to 83%, and 64% to 75% for diagnostic testing recommendations, recommendations for medical therapy, and recommendations for clinic-based therapy, respectively. A smaller study,[53] limited to suspected neoplasms, found 92% agreement on the decision to biopsy. Two other studies reported κ values for the dichotomous management outcome of "refer versus not refer" of 0.92[55] and 0.83.[54]

Several studies compared management agreement between clinic dermatologists and teledermatologists. In a study of 49 patients who had pigmented lesions and skin neoplasms, clinic dermatologists and teledermatologists agreed on whether to biopsy the lesion in 100% of cases.[70] In another study, clinical dermatologists and teledermatologists agreed with each other regarding management plans in 65% of cases.[59] A separate study[51] found 90% management agreement between one clinic dermatologist and several teledermatologists who examined 29 patients. Another study[44] found significantly higher intragroup agreement among clinic dermatologists than agreement between clinic dermatologist and teledermatologist. Management plan agreement between clinic dermatologists and teledermatologists of 55% (51/92) was significantly worse than the intragroup agreement for clinic dermatologists (P = .0001). Pairwise comparison of six clinic dermatologists and six teledermatologists demonstrated agreement rates of 68% to 80%, 56% to 74%, and 63% to 70% for diagnostic testing recommendations, recommendations for medical therapy, and recommendations for clinic-based therapy, respectively.[38] For diagnostic testing recommendations, intragroup agreement for both teledermatologists and clinical dermatologists exceeded intergroup agreement. The investigators indicated that the disagreements between clinical dermatologists' and teledermatologists' management plans likely reflected differences in management style; the clinical dermatologists were primarily based at a Veteran's Affairs Medical Center and the teledermatologists were primarily based in an academic center or private practice.

DISCUSSION

Teledermatology demonstrated good performance in comparison to clinic-based consultation for diagnostic agreement and diagnostic accuracy. For diagnosis, teledermatologists agreed with each other and with clinic-based dermatologists at a rate comparable to intragroup agreement among clinic dermatologists. For clinical management, the conclusions are less convincing because of the few studies on the subject. Only one study[38] compared teledermatologist–clinic dermatologist pairs with clinic dermatologist–clinic dermatologist pairs for the same set of patients. That study found less agreement in management decisions for teledermatologist–clinic dermatologist pairs.

The need for improved access to dermatology care cannot be overstated. The most recent American Academy Dermatology Workforce Survey found that between 2002 and 2007, despite increases in the use of nonphysician clinicians employed in dermatology offices, average patient waiting times and demand for hiring of dermatologists showed only small changes. Female dermatologists, in particular, worked fewer total hours than male dermatologists.[79] Teledermatology (especially store-and-forward teledermatology) could tap into the female dermatology workforce and the retired dermatology workforce by providing a "work from home" option with flexible hours.

Before widespread implementation, however, we must identify situations where teledermatology works best. Although most of the published literature provides favorable evidence for teledermatology, studies are generally limited by small sample sizes and poorly defined outcomes. Different considerations apply to the use of teledermatology for certain skin conditions, especially rashes and neoplasms. First, different photography techniques may be needed. For example, distribution of the plaques of psoriasis on a patient's body may be more important than close-up details of a single plaque, whereas detailed close-ups and dermatoscopic images of a pigmented lesion may be critical for correct diagnosis. Second, outcomes should be defined differently for studies of rashes and neoplasms. Diagnostic agreement may be sufficient for eczematous conditions in which histopathology is not considered the gold standard (eg, differentiation of contact dermatitis from atopic dermatitis), whereas diagnostic accuracy is the most appropriate outcome for neoplasms (ie, histopathology is the gold standard for diagnosis of skin cancer). Third, although the management of rashes focuses primarily on disease control, the management of neoplasms hinges primarily on the decision as to whether or not to biopsy. Adequately powered studies for subgroups of skin conditions (especially rashes and neoplasms) with clearly defined outcomes are needed. Finally, under certain conditions, palpation may be critical for correct diagnosis (eg, differentiation of actinic keratoses from seborrheic dermatitis).[80,81]

The motivation and skill level of the referring physician,[82] imaging technician, and teledermatologist may all greatly impact outcomes. Although some referring physicians may welcome the advice of a dermatologist (especially in situations where no prior access has been available), in capitated health care systems, these recommendations may be perceived as simply "more work" for the primary care physician. In addition, the referring physician may be uncomfortable monitoring response to therapy or performing dermatologic procedures. In that case, teledermatology may only be able to function as a glorified triage mechanism, unless methods can be developed to provide education and support to primary care physicians. The level of training of the imaging technician could also dramatically impact outcomes. Some programs use a non–health

care employee (such as a secretary or photographer) for imaging and obtaining history, whereas other programs use nurses or physician extenders. Skilled imagers offer a greater potential for high-quality history, examination details (eg, palpation, microscopic examination of skin scrapings), or follow-up (eg, the ability to perform biopsies). However, the cost of the teledermatology program will increase proportionally with higher-skilled imagers. Finally, the expertise level of the teledermatologist may also be important, especially in the area of teledermatoscopy. The future of teledermatology may someday resemble the world of teleradiology, where subspecialized teleradiologists interpret only certain types of radiologic images. Although difficult to standardize, these "human factors" are critical to the success of any program and should be evaluated in future studies.

In summary, based on the results reported to date, teledermatology is a promising technique that may greatly benefit geographically isolated patients who would not otherwise be seen by a dermatologist, and may prove to decrease wait times for patients who are not geographically isolated by eliminating some unnecessary referrals for face-to-face consultation. Large randomized controlled trials using consistent measures of diagnostic agreement and diagnostic accuracy for a wide range of skin problems and specific types of skin conditions (eg, rashes versus neoplasms) will be necessary to quantify the benefits of teledermatology. This necessity is especially important in the area of skin neoplasms, where a missed melanoma may result in patient mortality. Additionally, more analyses of economic costs and benefits, patient and physician satisfaction, and the impact on treating underserved populations are important in understanding the potential usefulness of teledermatology in modern medicine.

REFERENCES

1. Jacobson CC, Resneck JS Jr, Kimball AB. Generational differences in practice patterns of dermatologists in the United States: implications for workforce planning. Arch Dermatol 2004;140(12): 1477–82.
2. Maguiness S, Searles GE, From L, et al. The Canadian Dermatology Workforce Survey: implications for the future of Canadian dermatology–who will be your skin expert? J Cutan Med Surg 2004;8(3): 141–7.
3. Tsang MW, Resneck JS Jr. Even patients with changing moles face long dermatology appointment wait-times: a study of simulated patient calls to

dermatologists. J Am Acad Dermatol 2006;55(1): 54–8.

4. Murphy RL Jr, Fitzpatrick TB, Haynes HA, et al. Accuracy of dermatologic diagnosis by television. Arch Dermatol 1972;105(6):833–5.

5. Grigsby B, Brown N. 1999 report on U.S. telemedicine activity. Portland (OR): Association of Telemedicine Service Providers; 2000.

6. Perednia DA. Telemedicine in dermatology: 21st century update. Dermatology Foundation Progress in Dermatology 2000;34(1):1–10.

7. Burdick AE, Hu S. 2003 Teledermatology Survey. American Telemedicine Association Meeting. May, 2004.

8. Mofid M, Nesbitt T, Knuttel R. The other side of teledermatology: patient preferences. J Telemed Telecare 2007;13(5):246–50.

9. Eminovic N, Witkamp L, de Keizer NF, et al. Patient perceptions about a novel form of patient-assisted teledermatology. Arch Dermatol 2006;142(5): 648–9.

10. Whited JD, Hall RP, Foy ME, et al. Patient and clinician satisfaction with a store-and-forward teledermatology consult system. Telemed J E Health 2004;10(4):422–31.

11. Demiris G, Speedie SM, Hicks LL. Assessment of patients' acceptance of and satisfaction with teledermatology. J Med Syst 2004;28(6):575–9.

12. Collins K, Walters S, Bowns I. Patient satisfaction with teledermatology: quantitative and qualitative results from a randomized controlled trial. J Telemed Telecare 2004;10(1):29–33.

13. Hicks LL, Boles KE, Hudson S, et al. Patient satisfaction with teledermatology services. J Telemed Telecare 2003;9(1):42–5.

14. Weinstock MA, Nguyen FQ, Risica PM. Patient and referring provider satisfaction with teledermatology. J Am Acad Dermatol 2002;47(1):68–72.

15. Williams TL, Esmail A, May CR, et al. Patient satisfaction with teledermatology is related to perceived quality of life. Br J Dermatol 2001;145(6):911–7.

16. Williams T, May C, Esmail A, et al. Patient satisfaction with store-and-forward teledermatology. J Telemed Telecare 2001;7(Suppl 1):45–6.

17. Loane MA, Bloomer SE, Corbett R, et al. Patient satisfaction with realtime teledermatology in Northern Ireland. J Telemed Telecare 1998;4(1):36–40.

18. Armstrong AW, Dorer DJ, Lugn NE, et al. Economic evaluation of interactive teledermatology compared with conventional care. Telemed J E Health 2007; 13(2):91–9.

19. Hockey AD, Wootton R, Casey T. Trial of low-cost teledermatology in primary care. J Telemed Telecare 2004;10(Suppl 1):44–7.

20. Whited JD, Datta S, Hall RP, et al. An economic analysis of a store and forward teledermatology consult system. Telemed J E Health 2003;9(4):351–60.

21. Loane MA, Oakley A, Rademaker M, et al. A cost-minimization analysis of the societal costs of realtime teledermatology compared with conventional care: results from a randomized controlled trial in New Zealand. J Telemed Telecare 2001;7(4):233–8.

22. Loane MA, Bloomer SE, Corbett R, et al. A randomized controlled trial assessing the health economics of realtime teledermatology compared with conventional care: an urban versus rural perspective. J Telemed Telecare 2001;7(2):108–18.

23. Loane MA, Bloomer SE, Corbett R, et al. A comparison of real-time and store-and-forward teledermatology: a cost-benefit study. Br J Dermatol 2000; 143(6):1241–7.

24. Bergmo TS. A cost-minimization analysis of a real-time teledermatology service in northern Norway. J Telemed Telecare 2000;6(5):273–7.

25. Jacklin P, Roberts J. Social cost-benefit analysis of teledermatology. Costs were understated. BMJ 2000;321(7265):896–7.

26. Oakley AM, Kerr P, Duffill M, et al. Patient cost-benefits of realtime teledermatology–a comparison of data from Northern Ireland and New Zealand. J Telemed Telecare 2000;6(2):97–101.

27. Wootton R, Bloomer SE, Corbett R, et al. Multicentre randomised control trial comparing real time teledermatology with conventional outpatient dermatological care: societal cost-benefit analysis. BMJ 2000; 320(7244):1252–6.

28. Loane MA, Bloomer SE, Corbett R, et al. Patient cost-benefit analysis of teledermatology measured in a randomized control trial. J Telemed Telecare 1999;5(Suppl 1):S1–3.

29. American Telemedicine Association telemedicine guidelines. Available at: http://atmeda.org/ICOT/teledermstandards.htm. Accessed October 26, 2008.

30. Pak H, Burg G. Store-and-forward teledermatology. Available at: http://www.emedicine.com/derm/TOPIC560.htm. Accessed October 26, 2008.

31. Cohen J. A coefficient of agreement for nominal scales. Educational and Psychological Measurement 1960;20:37–46.

32. Baba M, Seckin D, Kapdagli S. A comparison of teledermatology using store-and-forward methodology alone, and in combination with Web camera videoconferencing. J Telemed Telecare 2005;11(7): 354–60.

33. Pak HS, Harden D, Cruess D, et al. Teledermatology: an intraobserver diagnostic correlation study, part I. Cutis 2003;71(5):399–403.

34. Krupinski EA, LeSueur B, Ellsworth L, et al. Diagnostic accuracy and image quality using a digital camera for teledermatology. Telemed J 1999;5(3):257–63.

35. Taylor P, Goldsmith P, Murray K, et al. Evaluating a telemedicine system to assist in the management of dermatology referrals. Br J Dermatol 2001; 144(2):328–33.

36. Mahendran R, Goodfield MJ, Sheehan-Dare RA. An evaluation of the role of a store-and-forward teledermatology system in skin cancer diagnosis and management. Clin Exp Dermatol 2005;30(3):209–14.

37. Harrison PV, Kirby B, Dickinson Y, et al. Teledermatology–high technology or not? J Telemed Telecare 1998;4(Suppl 1):31–2.

38. Whited JD, Hall RP, Simel DL, et al. Reliability and accuracy of dermatologists' clinic-based and digital image consultations. J Am Acad Dermatol 1999;41(5 Pt 1):693–702.

39. Oztas MO, Calikoglu E, Baz K, et al. Reliability of Web-based teledermatology consultations. J Telemed Telecare 2004;10(1):25–8.

40. Kvedar JC, Edwards RA, Menn ER, et al. The substitution of digital images for dermatologic physical examination. Arch Dermatol 1997;133(2):161–7.

41. Du Moulin MF, Bullens-Goessens YI, Henquet CJ, et al. The reliability of diagnosis using store-and-forward teledermatology. J Telemed Telecare 2003;9(5):249–52.

42. Lyon CC, Harrison PV. A portable digital imaging system in dermatology: diagnostic and educational applications. J Telemed Telecare 1997;3(Suppl 1):81–3.

43. High WA, Houston MS, Calobrisi SD, et al. Assessment of the accuracy of low-cost store-and-forward teledermatology consultation. J Am Acad Dermatol 2000;42(5 Pt 1):776–83.

44. Bowns IR, Collins K, Walters SJ, et al. Telemedicine in dermatology: a randomised controlled trial. Health Technol Assess 2006;10(43):1–39, iii–iv, ix–xi.

45. Tucker WF, Lewis FM. Digital imaging: a diagnostic screening tool? Int J Dermatol 2005;44(6):479–81.

46. Chao LW, Cestari TF, Bakos L, et al. Evaluation of an Internet-based teledermatology system. J Telemed Telecare 2003;9(Suppl 1):S9–12.

47. Lewis K, Gilmour E, Harrison PV, et al. Digital teledermatology for skin tumours: a preliminary assessment using a receiver operating characteristics (ROC) analysis. J Telemed Telecare 1999;5(Suppl 1):S57–8.

48. Barnard CM, Goldyne ME. Evaluation of an asynchronous teleconsultation system for diagnosis of skin cancer and other skin diseases. Telemed J E Health 2000;6(4):379–84.

49. Rashid E, Ishtiaq O, Gilani S, et al. Comparison of store and forward method of teledermatology with face-to-face consultation. J Ayub Med Coll Abbottabad 2003;15(2):34–6.

50. Tait CP, Clay CD. Pilot study of store and forward teledermatology services in Perth, Western Australia. Australas J Dermatol 1999;40(4):190–3.

51. Zelickson BD, Homan L. Teledermatology in the nursing home. Arch Dermatol 1997;133(2):171–4.

52. Lim AC, Egerton IB, See A, et al. Accuracy and reliability of store-and-forward teledermatology: preliminary results from the St. George Teledermatology Project. Australas J Dermatol 2001;42(4):247–51.

53. Whited JD, Mills BJ, Hall RP, et al. A pilot trial of digital imaging in skin cancer. J Telemed Telecare 1998;4(2):108–12.

54. Moreno-Ramirez D, Ferrandiz L, Nieto-Garcia A, et al. Store-and-forward teledermatology in skin cancer triage: experience and evaluation of 2009 teleconsultations. Arch Dermatol 2007;143(4):479–84.

55. Moreno-Ramirez D, Ferrandiz L, Bernal AP, et al. Teledermatology as a filtering system in pigmented lesion clinics. J Telemed Telecare 2005;11(6):298–303.

56. Piccolo D, Smolle J, Wolf IH, et al. Face-to-face diagnosis vs telediagnosis of pigmented skin tumors: a teledermoscopic study. Arch Dermatol 1999;135(12):1467–71.

57. Massone C, Hofmann-Wellenhof R, Ahlgrimm-Siess V, et al. Melanoma screening with cellular phones. PLoS ONE 2007;2(5):e483.

58. Fabbrocini G, Balato A, Rescigno O, et al. Telediagnosis and face-to-face diagnosis reliability for melanocytic and non-melanocytic 'pink' lesions. J Eur Acad Dermatol Venereol 2008;22(2):229–34.

59. Loane MA, Corbett R, Bloomer SE, et al. Diagnostic accuracy and clinical management by realtime teledermatology. Results from the Northern Ireland arms of the UK Multicentre Teledermatology Trial. J Telemed Telecare 1998;4(2):95–100.

60. Loane MA, Gore HE, Corbett R, et al. Preliminary results from the Northern Ireland arms of the UK Multicentre Teledermatology Trial: effect of camera performance on diagnostic accuracy. J Telemed Telecare 1997;3(Suppl 1):73–5.

61. Gilmour E, Campbell SM, Loane MA, et al. Comparison of teleconsultations and face-to-face consultations: preliminary results of a United Kingdom multicentre teledermatology study. Br J Dermatol 1998;139(1):81–7.

62. Nordal EJ, Moseng D, Kvammen B, et al. A comparative study of teleconsultations versus face-to-face consultations. J Telemed Telecare 2001;7(5):257–65.

63. Oakley AM, Astwood DR, Loane M, et al. Diagnostic accuracy of teledermatology: results of a preliminary study in New Zealand. N Z Med J 1997;110(1038):51–3.

64. Lowitt MH, Kessler II, Kauffman CL, et al. Teledermatology and in-person examinations: a comparison of patient and physician perceptions and diagnostic agreement. Arch Dermatol 1998;134(4):471–6.

65. Lesher JL Jr, Davis LS, Gourdin FW, et al. Telemedicine evaluation of cutaneous diseases: a blinded comparative study. J Am Acad Dermatol 1998;38(1):27–31.

66. Phillips CM, Burke WA, Shechter A, et al. Reliability of dermatology teleconsultations with the use of

teleconferencing technology. J Am Acad Dermatol 1997;37(3 Pt 1):398–402.

67. Phillips CM, Burke WA, Allen MH, et al. Reliability of telemedicine in evaluating skin tumors. Telemed J 1998;4(1):5–9.

68. Loane MA, Gore HE, Bloomer SE, et al. Preliminary results from the Northern Ireland arms of the UK Multicentre Teledermatology Trial: is clinical management by realtime teledermatology possible? J Telemed Telecare 1998;4(Suppl 1):3–5.

69. Piccolo D, Smolle J, Argenziano G, et al. Teledermoscopy–results of a multicentre study on 43 pigmented skin lesions. J Telemed Telecare 2000;6(3): 132–7.

70. Shapiro M, James WD, Kessler R, et al. Comparison of skin biopsy triage decisions in 49 patients with pigmented lesions and skin neoplasms: store-and-forward teledermatology vs face-to-face dermatology. Arch Dermatol 2004;140(5):525–8.

71. Ferrandiz L, Moreno-Ramirez D, Nieto-Garcia A, et al. Teledermatology-based presurgical management for nonmelanoma skin cancer: a pilot study. Dermatol Surg 2007;33(9):1092–8.

72. Piccolo D, Soyer HP, Chimenti S, et al. Diagnosis and categorization of acral melanocytic lesions using teledermoscopy. J Telemed Telecare 2004; 10(6):346–50.

73. Lozzi GP, Soyer HP, Massone C, et al. The additive value of second opinion teleconsulting in the management of patients with challenging inflammatory, neoplastic skin diseases: a best practice model in dermatology? J Eur Acad Dermatol Venereol 2007;21(1):30–4.

74. Bauer P, Cristofolini P, Boi S, et al. Digital epiluminescence microscopy: usefulness in the differential diagnosis of cutaneous pigmentary lesions. A statistical comparison between visual and computer inspection. Melanoma Res 2000;10(4):345–9.

75. Jolliffe VM, Harris DW, Whittaker SJ. Can we safely diagnose pigmented lesions from stored video images? A diagnostic comparison between clinical examination and stored video images of pigmented lesions removed for histology. Clin Exp Dermatol 2001;26(1):84–7.

76. Piccolo D, Soyer HP, Burgdorf W, et al. Concordance between telepathologic diagnosis and conventional histopathologic diagnosis: a multiobserver store-and-forward study on 20 skin specimens. Arch Dermatol 2002;138(1):53–8.

77. Blum A, Hofmann-Wellenhof R, Luedtke H, et al. Value of the clinical history for different users of dermoscopy compared with results of digital image analysis. J Eur Acad Dermatol Venereol 2004; 18(6):665–9.

78. Braun RP, Meier M, Pelloni F, et al. Teledermatoscopy in Switzerland: a preliminary evaluation. J Am Acad Dermatol 2000;42(5 Pt 1):770–5.

79. Kimball AB, Resneck JS Jr. The US dermatology workforce: a specialty remains in shortage. J Am Acad Dermatol 2008;59(5):741–5.

80. Cox NH. Palpation of the skin–an important issue. J R Soc Med 2006;99(12):598–600.

81. Cox NH. A literally blinded trial of palpation in dermatologic diagnosis. J Am Acad Dermatol 2007;56(6):949–51.

82. Grigsby B, Brega AG, Bennett RE, et al. The slow pace of interactive video telemedicine adoption: the perspective of telemedicine program administrators on physician participation. Telemed J E Health 2007;13(6):645–56.

Consumer Empowerment in Dermatology

Heather E. Hoch, MS[a], Kristine L. Busse, MS[b],
Robert P. Dellavalle, MD, PhD, MSPH[a,c,d],*

KEYWORDS

- Health care consumer • Internet • Patient advocacy
- Medical information

WHAT IS A MEDICAL CONSUMER?

Increasing political pressure and improved access to medical information provided by the Internet have strengthened consumer (ie, patient and patient advocate) participation in the medical enterprise.[1] Advocates argue that consumer involvement helps research to better reflect patient needs and improves medical outcomes,[2] and major policy decisions to increasingly focus on patient-centered ideals.[3] Skeptics assert that unreliable sources may more easily influence patients.

Currently consumer resources focus on severe or potentially fatal diseases, such as heart disease, cancer, diabetes, and AIDS. The scarcity of dermatology advocacy may reflect the perception that many skin disorders seldom cause death.[4] Dramatic examples of life-threatening skin disease, such as metastatic melanoma,[5] however, do exist. Furthermore, many common skin conditions have significant morbidity resulting from the psychologic burden produced by visible disease manifestations. Psoriasis patients feel socially stigmatized,[6] and acne patients often suffer a "greater psychologic burden than a variety of other disparate chronic disorders."[7] The mental health of dermatology disease sufferers can deteriorate[8] even to the point of suicide.[9] More dermatology advocacy will help patients obtain better disease information and management.

CONSUMER SUCCESS IN OTHER FIELDS

AIDS provides the epitomal example of how consumer activism can change health care, especially for those who have a highly stigmatized diagnosis. Using methods ranging from red ribbons to civil disobedience, AIDS consumers have demonstrated how to creatively advocate for their cause.[10]

Cancer consumer groups also have increased in number[11] and influence in recent years.[12] Over the past decade, breast cancer has become the premier force in consumer-driven research, leading to the United States National Breast Cancer Coalition (NBCC) named as "the world's most influential medical consumer lobby group."[13] Breast cancer consumers now play a major role in research funding decisions and policy-making. The NBCC has

Supported by the University of Colorado Denver School of Medicine, Colorado Health Informatics Collaboration interdisciplinary academic enrichment funds (RPD), and by National Cancer Institute grant K-07 CA92550 (RPD). Student fellowship funding (HEH) provided by the University of Colorado Denver and the Cancer League of Colorado.

[a] Department of Dermatology, University of Colorado Denver School of Medicine, Mail Stop F-8127, P.O. Box 6511, Aurora, CO 80045, USA

[b] Department of Dermatology, Wright State University Boonshoft School of Medicine, 3640 Colonel Glenn Highway, Dayton, OH 45435, USA

[c] Dermatology Service, Department of Veterans Affairs Medical Center, 1055 Clermont Street, Mail Code 165, Denver, CO 80220, USA

[d] Colorado School of Public Health, 13001 E. 17th Place, Campus Box B119, Aurora, CO 80045, USA

* Corresponding author. Colorado School of Public Health, 13001 E. 17th Place, Campus Box B119, Aurora, CO, 80045.

E-mail address: robert.dellavalle@ucdenver.edu (R.P. Dellavalle).

Dermatol Clin 27 (2009) 177–183
doi:10.1016/j.det.2008.11.002

led a grassroots advocacy campaign to encourage the United States Congress to pass the Breast Cancer and Environmental Research Act, which would make peer-reviewed National Institutes of Health grants available to study the relationship between environmental factors and breast cancer.[14] The NBCC also has initiated Project LEAD (leadership, education, and advocacy development) that provides scientific training to breast cancer advocates and addresses the criticism that consumers lack the knowledge needed to influence research decisions.[15] The NBCC has brought "acceptance of the idea that breast cancer survivors must have a say when policies are formed and decisions about research funding are made."[15]

The Susan G. Komen for the Cure has "pioneered cause-related marketing" with pink ribbon campaigns that have raised awareness and funding.[16] Breast cancer advocates involved politicians and celebrities to widen their audience. The availability of "pink" products that promise to donate funds to breast cancer research gives all consumers, not only breast cancer advocates, the opportunity to promote breast cancer research funding. Pink ribbons serve as "a public education vehicle that lends instant recognition and a positive tone to an otherwise anxiety provoking issue."[17]

Prostate cancer advocacy also has increased and provided patients who have prostate cancer with decision-making tools to better weigh treatment risks and benefits.[1,18,19] These interventions have helped men take a more active role in treatment decisions,[1,18] decrease anxiety,[18] and increase knowledge of treatment side effects.[1]

RECENT TRENDS: DIRECT ADVERTISING, COMPLEMENTARY MEDICINE, CHILDHOOD VACCINE REFUSAL

Consumers clearly play an important role in driving the market for the medical services they receive. Annually, billions of dollars fund direct-to-consumer (DTC) pharmaceutical advertising.[20] Currently, approximately 5% of the United States population has received a prescription as a result of DTC advertising.[20] Although some believe that DTC advertising unduly preys on patient fears[12] and undermines the physician-patient relationship,[20] others believe it fosters physician-patient communication.[21–23]

On another front, the increased use of complementary and alternative medicine (CAM) illustrates consumer influence on health care delivery.[24] In studies in the United States and other developed nations, CAM use rates by cancer patients run from 7% to 73%[24,25] and cost of more than $36 billion dollars annually.[26] As a result of patient demand, many hospitals now offer CAM.[27] Governmental agencies (eg, National Center for Complementary and Alternative Medicine and the White House Commission on Complementary and Alternative Medicine Policy) also increasingly explore CAM efficacy.[28]

Although clinical research may be industry-driven, researcher-focused, and unresponsive to patient needs,[2,15,29] consumers serve as the ultimate recipients of research benefits,[2,15,29–32] and their contributions highlight their growing importance.[29,33] Mass media may further complicate consumer disease management decisions by publicizing breaking research with potentially misleading headlines.[34–36]

The importance of consumer influence is further demonstrated in the debate over childhood vaccines. Some parents remain reluctant to vaccinate their children because of a presumed link between vaccination and autism.[37] Despite the lack of a "causal association between measles mumps rubella (MMR) vaccine or thimerisol containing vaccines (TCVs) and autism,"[38] autism advocacy groups continue to campaign against vaccinating children. As a result of the vast consumer response, Sensible Action For Ending Mercury-Indcued Neurological Disorders (SafeMinds) has sponsored more than $750,000 in research in this area.[39] The strength of the autism advocacy movement has raised concern that large amounts of money for autism research have diverted funds away from other childhood diseases with less powerful advocacy groups.[40]

Researchers increasingly consult with consumers on scientific study design.[41] The Cochrane Skin Group (CSG) serves as an example of the growing inclusion of consumers in all levels of health care research. The CSG produces and disseminates systematic reviews of dermatologic practices. It routinely involves consumers in the production of systematic reviews of the medical literature.[42] Consumers serve as authors, translators, and reviewers.[43] Medical professionals have been encouraged by the CSG to make research more productive and relevant through alliances with consumers.[15] At the same time, medical journals have been challenged to involve patients through comment on their publications.[29]

Although critics air concerns,[44] many investigators cite examples of consumers improving all stages of trial design from establishing priorities and drafting experimental protocols to helping with recruitment and data analysis.[45] Consumers add enthusiasm, inject humanity into research teams, and offer clarity to medical writing by reducing jargon.[45] Further research should "identify whether their [consumer] involvement leads to actual, rather than merely perceived, benefits for research processes and output"[31] and examine associations between consumer involvement and changes in patient care.

THE INTERNET: NEW CHALLENGES AND OPPORTUNITIES

Consumers increasingly turn to the Internet for health information. In 2006, 113 million Americans searched for health-related information online,[46] but 75% of those who seek health information online do not consistently assess its validity or online posting date.[46] Governmental and nongovernmental agencies have responded with programs designed to fairly label reliable health information on the Internet. Alternative stamps of approval for Web sites that contain information deemed safe and useful for consumers have emerged after the failure of the World Health Organization's initiative to create a top-level Uniform Resource Locator (URL) Internet domain—"health"—that would include only verified information.[47] Sites, such as Healthfinder, MedlinePlus, and Health on the Net (HON), specify criteria that identify valid health information.[48]

Google has established an advisory group on health care, composed of representatives from consumer, physician, and provider organizations to help solve the problem of consumer misinformation.[49] When using the search engine, Google, clicking on the "For patients" link narrows the search toward sites that have been labeled by health information quality agencies. For example, using the search term, "acne" (Fig. 1), and clicking on the "For patients" link returns results frequently labeled by HON, the National Library of Medicine (NLM), and the Centers for Disease Control. HON "promotes and guides the deployment of useful and reliable online health information, and its appropriate and efficient use" and is accredited by the United Nations in Geneva.[50] Web sites, such as HON, emphasize the importance of users patrolling the sites that display the HONcode and alerting them of dubious content.[48]

Google has attempted to "enlist the help of the health community [organizations such as the NLM and HON] to help us know which links contain medically reliable information, sift these reliable links so that they tend to show up relatively earlier in the search results, and then let you [the consumer] decide which groups in the health community you trust."[51] Consumers, however, may fail to discern the stamps of approval on relevant medial information. Even when patients become critical of health information sites, the difficulty of

sifting through the abundance of material generated by an Internet search engine remains.

Although consumers may enter symptoms into search engines to obtain diagnoses,[52] physicians may benefit even more from this exercise.[53] Two physicians recently demonstrated that Google yielded correct diagnosis in 15 of 26 (58%) medical scenarios. Google was "exceedingly good at finding documents with co-occurrence of the signs and symptoms used as search terms and human experts are efficient in selecting relevant documents."[53]

In 1998, the most prevalent dermatology diagnosis was acne vulgaris—a disease which affects more than 80% of persons by age 21.[54,55] A Google search for "acne" led to many Web sites initiated by acne sufferers, health professionals, governmental agencies, and the public (eg, Wikipedia) (see Fig. 1). Many advertising Web sites claimed to offer patients the increased ability to manage and understand their skin condition. The results page offered a refined search for information on acne treatment, symptoms, tests and diagnosis, causes and risk factors, and advice for patients and health professionals. Nine of 13 immediate hits obtained from a search for "acne" were sponsored advertisements (see Fig. 1). It may be difficult for the average dermatologic consumer to differentiate such advertisements from unsponsored information.

Google has embraced the consumer-directed medical information search strategy and created multiple avenues for patients to access quality medical information on the Internet. For instance, of the top 10 dermatology diagnoses,[54] seven had the "For Patients" option on the initial Google search. In addition, there is a new information filtering option, DermSearch,[56] for dermatology patients searching for peer-reviewed information online. DermSearch, powered by Google, offers information from peer-reviewed medical sites to increase consumer education and awareness.

In addition to providing peer-reviewed information to consumers, tools, such as DermSearch, may shield patients from advertising. Using the search term, "psoriasis", on Google (using the "For patients" link) compared with DermSearch yields noticeably different results. Although the initial search results arguably are similar on both domains, the regular Google search yields an additional 10 sponsored links ranging from psoriasis.org to multiple Web sites hawking herbal remedies. A Google search for "melanoma more: for_patients" also raised concern. Among the sponsored sites was a Web site claiming, "the truth is that the proven cancer prevention strategies and

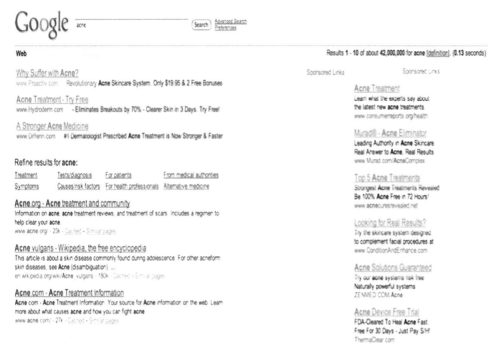

Fig. 1. Internet search from August 2008 of www.Google.com for "acne". (*Courtesy of* Google, Inc., Mountain View, CA.)

the real cures for cancer do not need a prescription, nor do they require surgery or barbaric procedures like radiation or chemotherapy."[57]

DERMATOLOGY CONSUMERS

Dermatology consumers may seek more Internet advice than other medical consumers because dermatologists spend less time with their patients on average than other physicians.[58] Frustration with the explanation received from a treating physician, feelings of helplessness, desire for anonymity, coping with feeling ill-informed, and seeking information for another all may be motivations for searching for online information.[59] Dermatologists, therefore, should attempt to guide their patients toward the most reputable sites of outside information possible.

In many practices, patients now can use e-mail communication to solicit information from their physicians or other members of the health care team to learn more about their specific conditions. The availability of e-mail as a new medium for information exchange allows for increased levels of consumer involvement in their own health care and also presents new challenges to physicians in terms of the efficiency, liability, and ethical responsibility of treating patients over the Web.

Physicians need assurance that patients will use e-mail privileges in an appropriate and resourceful manner. A recent study collected more than 3000

patient-physician e-mail messages to assess effectiveness. Results verified that the majority of e-mails focused on a single issue, with the most common topics relating to information updates for the physician, prescription renewals, questions about general health, obtaining test results, referrals, notes of gratitude or apology, and billing questions.[60] Perhaps more importantly, few e-mail conversations sought sensitive information, less than half required a physician response, and almost none transferred an urgent message.[60] The results suggest that patients benefit from communicating with their physicians by e-mail.

Additionally, 98% of patients were "very satisfied" with e-mail conversations and 65% of patients would more likely choose a physician who accepted e-mail.[61] Telephone volume of offices that implemented physician-patient e-mail services was 18.2% lower than offices that did not,[62] and answering patient questions by e-mail was 57% faster than by telephone.[63] Consumer-driven preferences will increase health care efficiency and optimize the physician-patient relationship. Although e-mail increases physician and patient communication, dermatologists also must consider patient health literacy.[19] Plain language information and decision aids should be available for all medical consumers[1] and must be implemented into areas of medical research. In response to this demand, some hospitals have librarians who conduct Internet searches and consolidate information packets for patients who have complex or rare medical issues.[64]

To facilitate the open exchange of medically relevant information, dermatology advocacy groups should moderate Web sites that help filter patient information. The National Psoriasis Foundation (NPF)[65] serves as a prime example—containing resources for patients regarding new developments in psoriasis research, providing information on treatment, and assisting patients with their search for a local physician. As a result, patients who are NPF members are more satisfied with the treatment they receive.[66]

SUMMARY

Health care consumers increasingly confront and collaborate with medical providers. This article describes recent developments in health care consumer activism including dermatology disease advocacy and efforts to improve dermatologist-patient interactions.

ACKNOWLEDGMENTS

The authors thank Greg Seitz, Avanta Collier, Carrie Cera Hill, Scott R. Freeman, Shayla O. Francis, Daniel Jensen, Hilda Bastien, Adam Asarch, and Kristie McNealy for comments on the manuscript.

REFERENCES

1. Holmes-Rovner M, Stableford S, Fagerlin A, et al. Evidence-based patient choice: a prostate cancer decision aid in plain language. BMC Med Inform Decis Mak 2005;5(16).
2. Tallon D, Chard J, Dieppe P. Consumer involvement in research is essential. BMJ 2000;320:380–1.
3. Calman K, Hine D. A policy framework for commissioning cancer services: a report by the expert advisory group on cancer to the chief medical officers of England and Wales. Available at: http://www.dh.gov.uk/prod_consum_dh/idcplg?IdcService=GET_FILE&dID=17110&Rendition=Web; 1995; Accessed June 27, 2007.
4. Stankler L. The effect of psoriasis on the sufferer. Clin Exp Dermatol 1981;3:303–6.
5. Bedikian AY, Johnson MM, Warneke CL, et al. Prognostic factors that determine the long-term survival of patients with unresectable metastatic melanoma. Cancer Invest 2008;26(6):624–33.
6. Weiss SC, Kimball AB, Liewehr DJ, et al. Quantifying the harmful effect of psoriasis on health-related quality of life. J Am Acad Dermatol 2002;47(4):512–8.
7. Dreno B. Assessing quality of life in patients with acne vulgaris. Am J Clin Dermatol 2006;7(2):99–106.
8. Gupta M, Gupta A. Depression and suicidal ideation in dermatology patients with acne, alopecia areata, atopic dermatitis and psoriasis. Br J Dermatol 1998;139(5):846–50.
9. Cotterill JA, Cunliffe WJ. Suicide in dermatological patients. Br J Dermatol 1997;137:246–50.
10. Sepkowitz KA. AIDS–the first 20 years. N Engl J Med 2001;344:1764–72.
11. Stevens T, Wilde D, Hunt J, et al. Overcoming the challenges to consumer involvement in cancer research. Health Expect 2003;6:81–8.
12. Williams-Jones B. 'Be ready against cancer, now': direct-to-consumer advertising for genetic testing. New Genet Soc 2006;25(1):89–107.
13. Anonymous. How consumers can and should improve clinical trials. Lancet 2001;357:1721.
14. National Breast Cancer Coalition. Grassroots advocacy 2007. Available at: http://www.natlbcc.org/bin/index.asp?strid=546&depid=5&btnid=0. Accessed June 27, 2007.
15. Liberati A. Consumer participation in research and health care. BMJ 1997;315:499.
16. Komen Breast Cancer Foundation: message from our founder. Available at: http://cms.komen.org/komen/AboutUs/MessageFromOurFounder/index.htm. Accessed September 21, 2008.
17. Vineburgh NT. The power of the pink ribbon: raising awareness of the mental health implications of terrorism. Psychiatry 2004;67(2):137–46.
18. Davison BJ, Degner LF. Empowerment of men newly diagnosed with prostate cancer. Can Nurse 1997;20(3):187–96.
19. Kim SP, Knight SJ, Tomori C, et al. Health literacy and shared decision making for prostate cancer patients with low socioeconomic status. Cancer Invest 2001;19(7):684–91.
20. Statement of the American College of Physicians for the Record of the Public Hearing on Consumer-Directed Promotion of Regulated Medical Products: Department of Health and Human Services Food and Drug Administration. Available at: http://www.acponline.org/hpp/dtc_fda.pdf. 2005. Accessed June 26, 2007.
21. Abel GA, Lee SJ, Weeks JC. Direct-to-consumer advertising in oncology: a content analysis of print media. J Clin Oncol 2007;25:1267–71.
22. Gellad ZF, Lyles KW. Direct-to-consumer advertising of pharmaceuticals. Am J Med 2007;120:475–80.
23. Viale PH, Yamamoto DS. The attitudes and beliefs of oncology nurse practitioners regarding direct-to-consumer advertising of prescription medications. Oncol Nurs Forum 2004;31(4):777–84.
24. Ernst E, Cassileth BR. The prevalence of complementary/alternative medicine in cancer: a systematic review. Cancer 1998;83:777–82.
25. Shen J, Andersen R, Albert PS, et al. Use of Complementary/alternative therapies by women with

advanced-stage breast cancer. BMC Complement Altern Med 2002;2(8).

26. Clement JP, Hsueh-Fen C, Burke D. Are consumers reshaping hospitals? Complementary and alternative medicine in US hospitals, 1999–2003. Health Care Manage Rev 2006;31(2):109–18.

27. Larson L. Natural selection: weaving complementary medicine into your health system. Trustee 2001; 54(4):6–12.

28. White house commission on complementary and alternative medicine policy final report 2002. Available at: http://www.whccamp.hhs.gov/. Accessed September 21, 2008.

29. Goodare H, Lockwood S. Involving patients in clinical research. Improves the quality of research. BMJ 1999;319:724–5.

30. Phillips WR, Grams GD. Involving patients in a primary care research meeting worked well. BMJ 2003;326:1329.

31. Hanley B, Truesdale A, King A, et al. Involving consumers in designing, conducting, and interpreting randomised controlled trials: questionnaire survey. BMJ 2001;322:519–23.

32. Smith R. The trouble with medical journals. London: RSM Press; 2006.

33. McCormick S, Brody J, Brown P, et al. Public involvement in breast cancer research: an analysis and model for future research. Int J Health Serv 2004;34:625–46.

34. Chabner BA, Kaufman D. Pity the poor consumer. Oncologist 2002;7:475–6.

35. American Urological Association. New study strengthens association of prostate cancer with exposure to agent orange sciencedaily. Available at: http://www.sciencedaily.com/releases/2008/05/080515072810.htm. 2008. Accessed August 4, 2008.

36. Public Library of Science. Eating broccoli may keep prostate cancer away, study suggests. Sciencedaily. Available at: http://www.sciencedaily.com/releases/2008/07/080701221450.htm. 2008; Accessed August 4, 2008.

37. Murch SH, Anthony A, Casson DH, et al. Retraction of an interpretation. Lancet 2004;363(9411):750.

38. DeStefano F. Vaccines and autism: evidence does not support a causal association. Clin Pharmacol Ther 2007;82(6):756–9.

39. Safeminds: about us. Available at: http://www.safeminds.org/home/about.html. Accessed September 21, 2008.

40. Anonymous. Clinical precision. Nature 2007;448(7154):623–4.

41. Boote J, Telford R, Cooper C. Consumer involvement in health research: a review and research agenda. Health Policy 2002;61:213–36.

42. Collier A, Johnson KR, Delamere F, et al. The Cochrane skin group: promoting the best evidence. J Cutan Med Surg 2005;9:324–31.

43. Collier A, Johnson K, Heilig L, et al. A win-win proposition: fostering US health care consumer involvement in the Cochrane collaboration skin group. J Am Acad Dermatol 2005;53:920–1.

44. Williamson C. What does involving consumers in research mean? QJM 2001;94:661–4.

45. Paterson C. How to involve consumers in your research team. Complement Ther Med 2005;13:61–4.

46. Fox S. Pew Internet Report 2006. Available at: http://www.pewinternet.org/PPF/r/190/report_display.asp. Accessed September 21, 2008.

47. Brown P. WHO calls for a health domain name to help consumers. BMJ 2002;324(7337):566.

48. Adams S, de Bonte A. Information Rx: prescribing good consumerism and responsible citizenship. Health Care Anal 2007;15:273–90.

49. Porter S. Google taps health care experts for new advisory council. AAFP News Now: American Academy of Family Physicians. Available at. http://www.aafp.org/online/en/home/publications/news/news-now/inside-aafp/20060627googlecouncil.printerview.html. 2007; Accessed September 21, 2008.

50. Health on the Net. Subscribed links profile. Available at: http://www.google.com/coop/profile?user=005783327436231643349&leftnav=no_directory. Accessed September 21, 2008.

51. Bosworth Adam. How do you know you're getting the best care possible? Posted Mar 2007. Available at: http://googleblog.blogspot.com/2007/03/how-do-you-know-youre-getting-best-care.html. Accessed October 27, 2008.

52. Keselmen A, Browne A, Kaufman D. Consumer health information seeking as hypothesis testing. J Am Med Inform Assoc 2008;15(4):484–95.

53. Tang H, Hwee Kwoon Ng J. Googling for a diagnosis—use of Google as a diagnostic aid: internet based study. BMJ 2006;333(7579):1143–5.

54. Feldman SR, Fleischer AB, McConnell RC. Most common dermatologic problems identified by internists, 1990-1994. Arch Intern Med 1998;158:726–30.

55. Smithard A, Glazebrook C, Williams HC. Acne prevalence, knowledge about acne and psychological morbidity in mid-adolescence: a community-based study. Br J Dermatol 2001;145:274–9.

56. Huang SJ. Dermsearch. Available at: http://www.dermsearch.com. Accessed January 4, 2009.

57. Bollinger T. Cancer-step outside the box. Available at: http://www.cancertruth.net/?gclid=COyMvu7Q2ZUCFS-JlagodM29RWg. Accessed September 21, 2008.

58. Trends and indicators in the changing health care marketplace section 6: trends in health plan and provider relationships. Available at: http://www.kff.org/insurance/7031/print-sec6.cfm. Accessed September 21, 2008.

59. Eysenbach G, Diepgen TL. Patients looking for information on the internet and seeking teleadvice. Arch Dermatol 1999;135:151–6.

60. White CB, Mover CA, Stern DT, et al. A content analysis of email communication between patients and their providers: patients get the message. J Am Med Inform Assoc 2004;11(4):260–7.

61. Anand SG, Feldman MJ, Geller DS, et al. A content analysis of email communication between primary care providers and parents. Pediatrics 2005; 115(5):1283–8.

62. Liederman EM, Lee JC, Baquero VH, et al. Patient-physician web messaging. The impact on message volume and satisfaction. J Gen Intern Med 2005; 20(1):52–7.

63. Rosen P, Kwoh CK. Patient-physician email: an opportunity to transform pediatric health care delivery. Pediatrics 2007;120(4):701–6.

64. Volk RM. Expert searching in consumer health: an important role for librarians in the age of the Internet and the Web. J Med Libr Assoc 2007;95(2):203–7.

65. National Psoriasis Foundation. National Psoriasis Foundation. Available at: http://www.psoriasis.org. Accessed January 4, 2009.

66. Gordon KB. Patient education and advocacy groups: a means to better outcomes? Arch Dermatol 2005; 141:80–1.

Registry Research in Dermatology

Luigi Naldi, MD[a,c],*, Liliane Chatenoud, ScBiol[a,b]

KEYWORDS

- Epidemiology • Registry • Incidence • Prognosis
- Skin disease • Cancer • Mortality • Procedures

WHAT IS A REGISTRY?

In the most general terms, a medical "registry" can be defined as a "systematic collection of information on all the cases of a particular disease or other health relevant condition."[1] The term applies to the process of collecting data and to the final result of such a process (ie, the file or database containing the information, properly, the "register"). According to the setting from which cases are collected, one can distinguish hospital-based and population-based registries. A hospital-based registry contains data on patients who have a specific type of disease diagnosed and treated at a given hospital or network of hospitals.[2] A population-based registry contains records for people diagnosed with a specific type of disease who reside within a defined geographic region. For example, a hospital can contribute to a melanoma registry with records from melanoma cases treated at the hospital. The hospital-based registry would not include all the people who have melanoma in the community, because some people may go elsewhere for treatment. A population-based registry, conversely, would contain data on people who have melanoma and live in a certain area, regardless of where they receive their treatment. People who live outside the geographic area covered by the population-based registry would not be counted, even if they receive medical care at a facility within the area. Population-based registries must collect data from many sources to make sure that a maximal number of cases in the community are collected.

Cancer registries are well known,[3] but registries can also collect data on other acute or chronic conditions, such as diabetes, heart disease, stroke, dementia, or birth defects. Public health registries of communicable disease compel registration of the occurrence of selected infections.[4]

In addition to disease registries, there are several other types of registries. In most developed countries, births and deaths are recorded through birth and death registration systems. Twin registries enroll pairs of twins who accept participation in medical and scientific research.[5] Procedure registries contain information about persons undergoing a specific medical procedure, such as mammography or coronary artery bypass graft surgery. Treatment registries are implemented to understand prescription profiles and to assess effectiveness and safety of a new medication. Exposure registries contain information about individuals at high risk for disease because of exposure to hazardous substances in the workplace or environment. Registries of families whose members have higher prevalence of inherited diseases are also a form of exposure registry.

In addition population-based and hospital-based registries, Web-based registries are increasingly common.[6] Their status is difficult to define. Being based on voluntary contribution by Web site visitors, they are not truly population based. The final sample may be largely biased by factors affecting Internet use and willingness to contribute information.

At variance with other data collections in medical research, registries are usually not centered around

a Centro Studi Gruppo Italiano Studi Epidemiologici in Dermatologia (GISED), Ospedali Riuniti, Largo Barozzi 1, 24100 Bergamo, Italy
b Department of Epidemiology, Mario Negri Institute for Pharmacological Research, Milan, Italy
c Department of Dermatology, Ospedali Riuniti, Bergamo, Italy
* Corresponding author.
E-mail address: luigi.naldi@gised.it (L. Naldi).

Dermatol Clin 27 (2009) 185–191
doi:10.1016/j.det.2008.11.004

a single specific hypothesis. Instead, they should be considered monitoring instruments or hypothesis generating tools.

Hospital- and population-based registries serve different purposes. Hospital-based registries, which usually involve active follow-up of enrolled patients, focus on prognosis and effectiveness or cost-effectiveness of care, with the final aim of improving disease management.

Population-based registries, conversely, provide information about the occurrence (incidence) of a health condition and its demographics—in other words, its descriptive epidemiology and burden. Data from population-based registries may allow evaluation of the effectiveness of disease prevention or control programs.[7] Data collected in the context of population-based registries sometimes are correlated with exposure data on a population basis in "ecological correlations."[8]

ESSENTIAL REQUIREMENTS FOR A REGISTRY

Registries require (1) unambiguous definitions of cases, (2) thorough procedures to identify cases, (3) systematic methods for case registration that minimize missing data, and (4) standardized procedures for collecting and storing data and ensuring data confidentiality. Case definition is especially important in this context. Reliable criteria are required to classify cases. Unfortunately, formally developed diagnostic criteria with known sensitivity, specificity, and predictive values are available only for a limited number of conditions; most registries have to rely on empirically developed diagnostic criteria.

Case identification is also important. Even within the boundaries of a hospital, there are many places in which diagnoses of a target disorder may be made and documented. It is thus necessary to identify each of those sources and to arrange access to the appropriate records. For cases not definitely confirmed, a decision must be made as to which cases are to be included. Such a decision may be difficult when nonspecific terms, such as *probable*, *possible*, *consistent with*, and others, are a part of the final diagnosis.

Because a major task is to follow up patients, the concept of "class of case" has great importance in the context of hospital-based registries.[9] The class of case divides cases into categories to be included or not in survival statistics. The generally accepted definitions of the six classes of case are (1) diagnosed at the registry hospital since the reference (starting) date of the hospital registry and all the first course of therapy given elsewhere, (2) diagnosed and treated at the registry hospital, (3) diagnosed elsewhere but

received all or part of the first course of therapy at the registry hospital, (4) diagnosed and all the first course of therapy received elsewhere (this would include patients admitted for only supportive care), (5) diagnosed and treated at the registry hospital before the reference (starting) date of the hospital registry, and (6) diagnosed only at autopsy. Cases included in categories 1, 2, and 3 are generally referred to as "analytical cases," and all such cases are included in patient survival calculations.

In the planning of a population-based registry, accurate and regularly published population data, including population figures by gender and 5-year age group, are required for the registration area and for any subdivisions.

Reporting of cases to a registry may be voluntary or compulsory by legislation or administrative order. The legal aspects of disease registration must be considered when planning a registry: in many countries, it is necessary to ensure a legal basis for the registry and to consider the protection of individual privacy. It is paramount that the issue of confidentiality be taken into account.[10]

Statistic methods, such as the capture-recapture strategy originally developed by biologists to track wild animal populations, that involve comparison of data from several independent overlapping sample frames adjusting for missing cases may be used to estimate the actual size of the disease population, and hence the degree of population coverage by the registry.[11]

Items to be carefully considered when reading registry research are summarized in **Box 1**.

PECULIARITIES OF DERMATOLOGY

There are peculiarities of dermatology in terms of disease frequency, classification, and management, which may have relevant implications for registry studies. Unlike most other organs, which usually count approximately 50 to 100 diseases, the skin has a complement of 1500 to 2000 conditions.[12] In addition to disorders primarily affecting the skin, there are cutaneous manifestations with most of the major systemic diseases (eg, vascular and connective tissue diseases). The classification of skin disorders is far from satisfactory, with the widespread use of symptom-based or purely descriptive terms, such as *parapsoriasis*. For the dermatologist, the International Classification of Disease (ICD) coding system is a crude and cumbersome instrument full of inconsistencies. The recognition of the deficiencies prompted several initiatives, including the Diagnostic Index of the British Association of Dermatologists and the Diagnostic Index commissioned by the US

1. Is the registry "base" clearly specified (ie, population base versus hospital base versus less clearly defined bases)?
2. Is the registry health condition clearly defined (eg, disease versus procedure versus treatment)?
3. For disease registries, is a valid and repeatable disease definition given?
4. For disease registries, are the diagnostic criteria clearly identified and met by the patients included in the registry?
5. Are the procedures for identifying cases clearly presented?
6. Is information about registry coverage and completeness provided?
7. Are standardized procedures for collecting and storing data adopted and presented?
8. Are data security and confidentiality ensured?
9. For population-based registries, is the surveyed population clearly identified and are demographic data available?
10. For any specific analysis, are starting date and time interval of surveillance clearly presented?

National Institute for Arthritis and Musculoskeletal and Skin Diseases (NIAMS). These instruments may improve classification and communication but are not yet widely adopted.[13]

As a whole, skin diseases, including several varieties of skin cancer, are exceedingly common, and most dermatology occurs in the outpatient arena. In general, only a fraction of those individuals who have skin disease are expected to seek medical help. Conversely, severe skin disorders with an impact in terms of mortality, such as autoimmune bullous diseases, are rare, making their surveillance difficult.

REGISTRIES IN DERMATOLOGY

There are registries established in several areas of dermatology (**Table 1**). Here, the authors cover selected programs.

Cancer Registries

Accurate ascertainment is a problem for all cancers in population-based registries, but it is an overwhelming task for skin cancer.[14] Shortfalls in ascertainment for the diagnosis of skin cancer

have several sources, including increased use of outpatient treatment, lack of pathologic documentation, variability of diagnosis among individual pathologists, and use of private care. The need for specialized population-based skin cancer registries has been repeatedly considered.[15] One example of a specialized skin cancer registry is that of the Trentino province in northeast Italy, started in 1992.[16] Another example is the registration of nonmelanoma skin cancer in West Glamorgan, South Wales.[17] Ad hoc surveys for skin cancer may also be conducted within the framework of more general population-based cancer registries. Cancer registries intensively surveying for skin cancer are, among the others, the registry of the Swiss Cantons of Vaud and Neuchâtel, the Schleswig-Holstein registry in Germany, the Tuscany registry in Italy, the Southeastern Arizona Skin Cancer Registry, and the New South Wales Central Cancer Registry in Australia.[18–22] In addition to incidence data, analyses from these registries, if complemented with follow-up data, provide information on prognostic factors for survival and on the impact of early detection campaigns.[23] Specialized registries may have a particular value when assessing rare varieties of skin cancer, such as Merkel carcinoma, adnexal skin cancer, or sebaceous carcinoma.[24]

Registries of Rare Disorders

There is great opportunity in dermatology to establish hospital-based registries of rare disorders. The National Epidermolysis Bullosa Registry, based in Nashville, Tennessee, has provided relevant contributions to the classification of epidermolysis bullosa and to a better understanding of systemic involvement and complications.[25–27] The National Registry for Ichthyosis and Related Disorders at the University of Washington was created with the support of the National Institutes of Health (NIH) to encourage research into the diagnosis and treatment of ichthyoses and related disorders.[28] The National Alopecia Areata Registry, also funded by the NIH, has been a highly successful registry. Materials from this registry, including samples of DNA, lymphoblast lines, and sera, collected from well-characterized individuals, multiplex families, and sibling pairs have been the foundation of studies looking at susceptibility genes for alopecia areata by means of linkage analysis and genome-wide scan.[29]

Other examples of registries of rare disorders of interest to dermatologists are the registry of hereditary α_1-antitrypsin deficiency at the University of Leiden;[30] the French National Registry of

Table 1 Different types of registries, with examples in dermatology	
Type of Registry	Example in Dermatology
According to the base from which data are collected	
Population-based registry	Specialized skin cancer registries[16,17]
Hospital-based registry	The Regiscar program in Europe collecting data on severe cutaneous adverse reactions[39]
According to the condition being registered	
Disease registry	National Epidermolysis Bullosa Registry[25–27]
Procedure registry	Registries of skin complication in organ transplant recipients[43,45,46]
Treatment registry	Registries of systemic treatment for psoriasis (eg, Psocare program in Italy)[48–50]
Twin registry	Analyses from the Danish nationwide twin cohort on the heritability of psoriatic arthritis[52]

Childhood Hematological Malignancies, collecting cases of childhood Langerhans cell histiocytosis, at the Institut National de la Santé et de la Recherche Médicale (INSERM) in France;[31] and the National Epidemiologic Registry of Cryptococcosis at the National Reference Center for Mycoses in France.[32] Several hospital-based registries, mainly run by rheumatologists, consider rheumatologic disorders with particular skin manifestations, such as antiphospholipid syndrome in the pediatric population, subacute cutaneous lupus erythematosus, neonatal lupus, juvenile dermatomyositis, and systemic sclerosis.[33–37] The population-based registry of severe cutaneous adverse reaction coordinated by the Dokumentationzentrum schwerer Hautreationen of the University of Freiburg in Germany provides a prime example of a registry combined with additional research modules and integrated into a wider network. The registry has been complemented with case-control surveillance of risk factors for severe reactions and with a biologic data bank for pharmacogenetic studies. It has also been integrated into a wider European network sharing the same objectives, the Regiscar program.[38–40]

Registries may help to characterize and understand the etiology of newly described conditions. For example, data from the registry of nephrogenic systemic fibrosis (or nephrogenic fibrosing dermopathy), maintained at the Yale University, have pointed to a link between the disease and systemic administration of gadolinium-containing MRI contrast agents in patients with renal insufficiency.[41]

Registries may be implemented as part of pharmaceutical company marketing or promotional agendas. In contrast to the Web-based Fabry Registry, whose support from pharmaceutical companies is not openly disclosed on the Web,[42] registry sponsorship information should be openly disclosed.

If complemented with biologic data banks, registries of rare disorders may provide invaluable insights into genetic predisposition and pathophysiology. They may help to care for the patient by improving diagnostic criteria and by standardizing management.

Registries of Procedures

An area in which registries have been organized in several countries is skin complications in organ transplant recipients. The Israel Penn International Transplant Tumor Registry at the University of Cincinnati is the largest and most comprehensive transplant tumor registry in the world; however, it is not focused on skin cancer.[43] In consideration of the peculiarities of skin complications, including cosmetic changes, infection, and skin cancer, dermatology-based registries of patients who have undergone transplantation have been started in several countries. For example, a registry of major skin complications in patients who have received a renal, heart, or liver transplant since May 1969 was started in 1996 at several transplantation units in Italy.[44] Similar dermatology-based registries are active in The Netherlands, France, Germany, Ireland, and other countries. In addition to contributing estimates of the risk for skin cancer and other major skin complications (eg, deep cutaneous fungal infections) in transplant patients, these registries have improved patient education and skin care.[45] Data from several of these registries have been combined in the context of international collaborations, such as the Skin Care in Organ Transplant Patients Europe (SCOPE) initiative, or have been complemented with biologic data to throw light onto pathomechanisms, such as in the context of the HPV-UV-CA program aimed at assessing the role of infection by HPV in skin cancer.[46,47]

Treatment Registries

These registries are mainly implemented to assess safety and long-term effectiveness of newly developed treatments. For example, the limitations of premarketing data concerning so-called "biologic" agents for psoriasis have prompted the development of registries of systemic treatment for psoriasis in several different countries, mainly in Europe.[48] The Psocare project is a nationwide registry in Italy.[49] Psoriatic patients receiving a new systemic treatment for their condition for the first time in their life, including conventional and biologic agents, are eligible. Enrolled patients are followed up for a minimum period of 3 years after entry. The main focus is on factors influencing efficacy and on long-term safety. The registry is fully supported by the Italian Drug Agency, and a total of 152 reference centers for the treatment of moderate to severe psoriasis in Italy participate. Registries with similar aims are activated in other countries, for example, the PsoBest registry in Germany, the PsoReg registry in Sweden, the Biobadaser registry in Spain, and the Bid-BAD registry in the United Kingdom.[50] Recently, a collaboration among these different registries has been envisaged, and the Psonet international network has been started with the aim of combining data from national-based registries.[51] The Psonet collaboration fit well with the requirement of a Europe-wide proactive pharmacovigilance put forward by the European Drug Agency (EMEA), and was fostered with the establishment of the European Network of Pharmacovigilance and Pharmacoepidemiology Centres (ENCePP) under EMEA patronage. The Psonet collaboration has been invited to be part of such an EMEA network.[48]

Other Registry Experiences

There are examples of several other registry-based research activities in dermatology. In particular, twin registries offer invaluable insights into genetic-environmental interaction with estimates of heritability (ie, the proportion of phenotypic variation in a population that is attributable to genetic variation among individuals).[52,53] Heritability is an important measure to improve the understanding of the etiology of multifactorial diseases, such as psoriasis.[53]

ON THE HORIZON

With the increasing role of electronically based information management, the use of registries should increase in the near future. Registries could be integrated into a complex research framework. Record linkage that involves a combination of data from different sources allows facile hypotheses testing. Recent examples of these analyses are the assessment of cancer risk associated with ultraviolet light B phototherapy and with exposure to photosensitizing diuretics.[54,55] Banks of biologic materials can also be effectively combined with registries as a valuable resource for future basic research, such as searches for susceptibility genes.[56]

SUMMARY

Hospital- and population-based registries serve different purposes. A hospital-based registry mainly focuses on prognosis and effectiveness of care, whereas population-based registries mainly provide information about the incidence of a health condition. There are registries established in several areas of dermatology, including, among others, specialized population-based skin cancer registries; registries of rare disorders (eg, The National Epidermolysis Bullosa Registry); registries of skin complications in people undergoing specific procedures, such as organ transplantation; and treatment registries, such as those collecting data on systemic treatment for psoriasis grouped within the Psonet initiative in Europe. With the increasing role of electronic data storage and retrieval, the use of registries and their linkage analysis should increase.

FURTHER READINGS

International Agency of Cancer. http://www.iarc.fr/.
National Registry for Ichthyosis and Related Disorders. http://depts.washington.edu/ichreg/ichthyosis.registry/.
Alopecia Areata Registry. http://www.mdanderson.org/departments/alopecia/.
Israel Penn International Transplant Tumor Registry. http://www.ipittr.org/Home.htm.
Regiscar. http://regiscar.uni-freiburg.de/.
Psocare. http://www.psocare.it/cms/.
Psonet. http://www.psonet.eu/.
Australian Twin Registry. http://www.twins.org.au/index.php?page=0.

REFERENCES

1. Last JM. A dictionary of epidemiology. 4th edition. New York: Oxford University Press; 2001.

2. Roos LL, Nicol JP. A research registry: uses, development, and accuracy. J Clin Epidemiol 1999;52:39–47.

3. Parkin DM. The role of cancer registries in cancer control. Int J Clin Oncol 2008;13:102–11.

4. Judelsohn RG, Koslap-Petraco MB. Public health perspectives on the rising incidence of pertussis. Public Health Nurs 2007;24:421–8.

5. Ohm Kyvik K, Derom C. Data collection on multiple births—establishing twin registers and determining zygosity. Early Hum Dev 2006;82:357–63.

6. Krengel S, Breuninger H, Hauschild A, et al. Installation of a network for patients with congenital melanocytic nevi in German-speaking countries. J Dtsch Dermatol Ges 2008;6:204–8.

7. Saraiya M, Ahmed F, White M, et al. Toward using National Cancer Surveillance data for preventing and controlling cervical and other human papillomavirus-associated cancers in the US. Cancer 2008; 113(S10):2837–40.

8. Elliott P, Martuzzi M, Shaddick G, et al. Spatial statistical methods in environmental epidemiology: a critique. Stat Methods Med Res 1995;4:137–59.

9. Pession A, Dama E, Rondelli R, et al. Survival of children with cancer in Italy, 1989–98. A report from the hospital based registry of the Italian Association of Paediatric Haematology and Oncology (AIEOP). Eur J Cancer 2008;44:1282–9.

10. Ingelfinger JR, Drazen JM. Registry research and medical privacy. N Engl J Med 2004;350:1452–3.

11. Wang Y, Druschel CM, Cross PK, et al. Problems in using birth certificate files in the capture-recapture model to estimate the completeness of case ascertainment in a population-based birth defects registry in New York State. Birth Defects Res A Clin Mol Teratol 2006;76:772–7.

12. Stevens A, Raftery J, Mant J, et al. Health care needs assessment. The epidemiologically based needs assessment reviews. Third series. Oxford: Radcliffe Publishing Ltd; 2007.

13. Papier A, Chalmers RJG, Byrnes JA, et al. Framework for improved communication: the dermatology lexicon project. J Am Acad Dermatol 2004;50:630–4.

14. Brewster D, Coebergh J, Storm H, et al. Population-based cancer registries: the invisible key to cancer control. Lancet Oncol 2005;6:193–5.

15. Richards C, Richards H, Pheby D, et al. Skin cancer: how accurate are local data? BMJ 1995;310:503.

16. Boi S, Cristofolini M, Micciolo R, et al. Incidence and mortality data from cutaneous melanoma in Trentino: registry-based study. J Cutan Med Surg 2008;12: 59–63.

17. Holme SA, Malinovsky K, Roberts DL. Malignant melanoma in South Wales: changing trends in presentation (1986–98). Clin Exp Dermatol 2001;26:484–9.

18. Levi F, Randimbison L, Maspoli M, et al. High incidence of second basal cell skin cancers. Int J Cancer 2006;119:1505–7.

19. Katalinic A, Kunze U, Schäfer T. Epidemiology of cutaneous melanoma and non-melanoma skin cancer in Schleswig-Holstein, Germany: incidence, clinical subtypes, tumor stages and localization. Br J Dermatol 2003;149:1200–6.

20. Crocetti E, Carli P, Miccinesi G, et al. Melanoma incidence in central Italy will go on increasing also in the near future: a registry-based, age-period-cohort analysis. Eur J Cancer Prev 2007;16:50–4.

21. Harris RB, Griffith K, Moon TE, et al. Trends in the incidence of nonmelanoma skin cancers in southeastern Arizona, 1985–1996. J Am Acad Dermatol 2001;45:528–36.

22. Downing A, Yu XQ, Newton-Bishop J, et al. Trends in prognostic factors and survival from cutaneous melanoma in Yorkshire, UK and New South Wales, Australia between 1993 and 2003. Int J Cancer 2008;123:861–6.

23. Crocetti E, Mangone L, Lo Scocco G, et al. Prognostic variables and prognostic groups for malignant melanoma. The information from Cox and classification and regression trees analysis: an Italian population-based study. Melanoma Res 2006;16:429–33.

24. Dasgupta T, Wilson LD, Yu JB, et al. A retrospective review of 1349 cases of sebaceous carcinoma. Cancer 2008; [Epub ahead of print].

25. Fine JD, Eady RA, Bauer EA, et al. The classification of inherited epidermolysis bullosa (EB): report of the Third International Consensus Meeting on Diagnosis and Classification of EB. J Am Acad Dermatol 2008; 58:931–50.

26. Fine JD, Johnson LB, Weiner M, et al. Gastrointestinal complications of inherited epidermolysis bullosa: cumulative experience of the National Epidermolysis Bullosa Registry. J Pediatr Gastroenterol Nutr 2008; 46:147–58.

27. Fine JD, Hall M, Weiner M, et al. The risk of cardiomyopathy in inherited epidermolysis bullosa. Br J Dermatol 2008;159:677–82.

28. Ross R, DiGiovanna JJ, Capaldi L, et al. Histopathologic characterization of epidermolytic hyperkeratosis: a systematic review of histology from the National Registry for Ichthyosis and Related Skin Disorders. J Am Acad Dermatol 2008;59:86–90.

29. Martinez-Mir A, Zlotogorski A, Gordon D, et al. Genome-wide scan for linkage reveals evidence of several susceptibility loci for alopecia areata. Am J Hum Genet 2007;80:316–28.

30. Fregonese L, Stolk J. Hereditary alpha-1-antitrypsin deficiency and its clinical consequences. Orphanet J Rare Dis 2008;3:16.

31. Guyot-Goubin A, Donadieu J, Barkaoui M, et al. Descriptive epidemiology of childhood Langerhans cell histiocytosis in France, 2000–2004. Pediatr Blood Cancer 2008;51:71–5.

32. Neuville S, Dromer F, Morin O, et al. Primary cutaneous cryptococcosis: a distinct clinical entity. Clin Infect Dis 2003;36:337–47.

33. Avcin T, Cimaz R, Silverman ED, et al. Pediatric antiphospholipid syndrome: clinical and immunologic features of 121 patients in an international registry. Pediatrics 2008;122:e1100–7.

34. Clancy RM, Backer CB, Yin X, et al. Genetic association of cutaneous neonatal lupus with HLA class II and tumor necrosis factor alpha: implications for pathogenesis. Arthritis Rheum 2004;50:2598–603.

35. Popovic K, Nyberg F, Wahren-Herlenius M, et al. A serology-based approach combined with clinical examination of 125 Ro/SSA-positive patients to define incidence and prevalence of subacute cutaneous lupus erythematosus. Arthritis Rheum 2007;56:255–64.

36. Gunawardena H, Wedderburn LR, North J, et al. Clinical associations of autoantibodies to a p155/140 kDa doublet protein in juvenile dermatomyositis. Rheumatology (Oxford) 2008;47:324–8.

37. Hudson M, Taillefer S, Steele R, et al. Improving the sensitivity of the American College of Rheumatology classification criteria for systemic sclerosis. Clin Exp Rheumatol 2007;25:663–754–7.

38. Mockenhaupt M, Idzko M, Grosber M, et al. Epidemiology of staphylococcal scalded skin syndrome in Germany. J Invest Dermatol 2005;124:700–3.

39. Ziemer M, Wiesend CL, Vetter R, et al. Cutaneous adverse reactions to valdecoxib distinct from Stevens-Johnson syndrome and toxic epidermal necrolysis. Arch Dermatol 2007;143:711–6.

40. Lonjou C, Borot N, Sekula P, et al. A European study of HLA-B in Stevens-Johnson syndrome and toxic epidermal necrolysis related to five high-risk drugs. Pharmacogenet Genomics. 2008;18:99–107.

41. Cowper SE. Nephrogenic fibrosing dermopathy: the first 6 years. Curr Opin Rheumatol 2003;15:785–90.

42. Hopkin RJ, Bissler J, Banikazemi M, et al. Characterization of Fabry disease in 352 pediatric patients in the Fabry registry. Pediatr Res 2008;64:550–5.

43. Buell JF, Gross TG, Woodle ES, et al. Malignancy after transplantation. Transplantation 2005;80(2 Suppl): S254–64.

44. Naldi L, Fortina AB, Lovati S, et al. Risk of nonmelanoma skin cancer in Italian organ transplant recipients. A registry-based study. Transplantation 2000; 70:1479–84.

45. Stasko T, Brown MD, Carucci JA, et al. Guidelines for the management of squamous cell carcinoma in organ transplant recipients. Dermatol Surg 2004; 30(4 Pt 2):642–50.

46. Matin RN, Mesher D, Proby CM, et al. Melanoma in organ transplant recipients: clinicopathological features and outcome in 100 cases. Am J Transplant 2008;8:1891–900.

47. Bouwes Bavinck JN, Euvrard S, Naldi L, et al. EPI-HPV-UV-CA group. Keratotic skin lesions and other risk factors are associated with skin cancer in organ-transplant recipients: a case-control study in The Netherlands, United Kingdom, Germany, France, and Italy. J Invest Dermatol 2007;127:1647–56.

48. Nijsten T, Wakkee M. Psocare: Italy shows the way in postmarketing studies. Dermatology 2008;217: 362–4.

49. Naldi L, Addis A, Chimenti S, et al. Impact of body mass index and obesity on clinical response to systemic treatment for psoriasis. Evidence from the Psocare project. Dermatology 2008;217:365–73.

50. Schmitt-Egenolf M. PsoReg—the Swedish registry for systemic psoriasis treatment. The registry's design and objectives. Dermatology 2007;214: 112–7.

51. Lecluse LLA, Naldi L, Stern RS, et al. National registries of systemic treatment for psoriasis and the European "Psonet" initiative. Dermatology; [in press].

52. Millard TP, Bataille V, Snieder H, et al. The heritability of polymorphic light eruption. J Invest Dermatol 2000;115:467–70.

53. Pedersen OB, Svendsen AJ, Ejstrup L, et al. On the heritability of psoriatic arthritis. Disease concordance among monozygotic and dizygotic twins. Ann Rheum Dis 2008;67:1417–21.

54. Hearn RM, Kerr AC, Rahim KF, et al. Incidence of skin cancers in 3867 patients treated with narrow-band ultraviolet B phototherapy. Br J Dermatol 2008;159:931–5.

55. Jensen AØ, Thomsen HF, Engebjerg MC, et al. Use of photosensitising diuretics and risk of skin cancer: a population-based case-control study. Br J Cancer 2008;99:1522–8.

56. Lu LJ, Wallace DJ, Navarra SV, et al. Lupus registries: evolution and challenges. Semin Arthritis Rheum 2008; [Epub ahead of print].

Dermatology Internet Resources

Rachel N. Simmons, BS[a], Jeffrey I. Ellis, MD[b,c],
Robert P. Dellavalle, MD, PhD, MSPH[d,e,f],*

KEYWORDS

- Dermatology internet resources
- Open access dermatology journals • Visual Dx health
- JournalReview.org

Public health promotes disease awareness and prevention. Many dermatology Internet resources benefit public health by providing information on the diagnosis and treatment of skin conditions. Dermatologic public health issues including infections, nutritional deficiencies, the importance of sun protection, and early diagnosis of skin cancer.[1] The Internet reaches millions of people worldwide with information on these important topics such as the "ABCs of melanoma."

Internet-based tools are changing clinical dermatology. Time is limited, with an aging population keeping dermatology clinics booked months in advance and an average dermatologist seeing more than four patients per hour.[2] When patient care questions arise, physicians increasingly turn to the Internet rather to than journals and textbooks.[3] Major search engines, such as Google, are often the first place physicians go for information. Although Google searches are useful, casting such a wide net is inefficient, because the user must discern the credible sources from low-quality information.[3–5] There are a variety of freely available dermatologic image banks, databases, and educational materials on the Internet. Numerous organizations, journals, and academic institutions from around the world have Web sites in English that offer helpful tools, such as image quizzes and searchable databases.[6]

The Internet, however, is much more than just a database for finding diagnostic information, drug dosages, or relevant articles. The Internet has revolutionized the way in which scientists and clinicians communicate with each other and relay information to the public.[7] Examples of Web 2.0, a user-focused Internet-based technology that fosters communication and collaboration,[8] abound. One is the Wikis, which allows users to simultaneously edit and annotate content on a given Web site.[9] The open platform of Web 2.0 allows continual analysis, refinement, and sharing of information, which benefits scientists, clinicians, and patients.[10] Dermatologists frequently manage diseases in conjunction with other specialties, such as rheumatology, gastroenterology, or infectious disease. Clinical questions commonly arise, triggering consultations with other physicians with more expertise. The enhanced form of telecommunication inherent in Web 2.0 allows dermatologists to correspond and consult

Dr. Ellis is president of JournalReview.org. Dr. Dellavalle sits on the editorial board of BMC Dermatology and The Open Dermatology Journal, and chairs the advisory panel for JournalReview.org. He receives no compensation for this work.

a University of Florida College of Medicine, P.O. Box 100518, Gainesville, FL 32610, USA
b Department of Dermatology, State University of New York Downstate, USA
c Dermatological Surgery, North Shore/Long Island Jewish Hospital, Belaray Dermatology, 2 Patton Place, Plainview, NY 11803, USA
d Department of Veterans Affairs Medical Center, 1055 Clermont Street, #165, Denver, CO, USA
e Department of Dermatology, University of Colorado Denver, School of Medicine, PO Box 6510, Mail Stop F703, Aurora, Denver, CO 80045–0510, USA
f Colorado School of Public Health, 13001 E. 17th Place, Campus Box B119, Aurora, CO 80045, USA
* Corresponding author. Colorado School of Public Health, 13001 E. 17th Place, Campus Box B119, Aurora, CO, 80045.
E-mail address: robert.dellavalle@ucdenver.edu (R.P. Dellavalle).

Dermatol Clin 27 (2009) 193–199
doi:10.1016/j.det.2008.11.009

efficiently with specialists from around the world, thereby increasing collaboration but sparing the time and cost of bringing people together.[7]

Here, the authors list freely and easily accessible English-language Web sites with useful information about skin diseases. They performed Google and PubMed searches for relevant Web sites by using key phrases, such as "dermatology resources," "dermatology learning tools," and "evidence-based dermatology." They also searched Google for Web sites on common dermatologic conditions by entering key words, such as "psoriasis" and "tinea pedis." They excluded resources charging a fee but included some that required user registration.

Three tables present the results: clinical resources (**Table 1**); educational materials for patients, students, and physicians (**Table 2**); and evidence-based medicine (**Table 3**). Web site addresses and brief summaries about each source appear in each table. The authors highlight one source from each category by providing more details about the Web site and how it could benefit dermatologists.

CLINICAL RESOURCES: OPEN ACCESS DERMATOLOGY JOURNALS

Patient care–related questions frequently arise from gaps in webs of medical knowledge.[11] New online dermatology journals such as *BMC Dermatology* and *The Open Dermatology Journal* are increasing the scholarly dermatology content on the Internet. The open-access movement encourages immediate online sharing of publicly funded research for the benefit of science, medicine, and society.[1] Studies have confirmed that open-access articles reach more readers than those requiring a subscription.[12] Increased readership may enrich knowledge, create new questions, and accelerate research as the writers of the open-access initiative envisioned.

Traditional subscription-based dermatology journals are also increasing free access to select articles to comply with the National Institute of Health (NIH) Public Access Policy. This policy mandates that all NIH funded peer-reviewed manuscripts accepted for publication become accessible to the public no later than 12 months after publication.[13] Authors who wish to accelerate this process can consider self-archiving, author posting of manuscripts on the Web.[14]

EDUCATIONAL MATERIALS: WWW.VISUALDXHEALTH.COM

The Internet makes medical information readily available, and health care consumers commonly research personal health problems online.[15] Last year, 56% of American adults sought information on a medical condition, with most using online resources.[16] Visual Dx Health is an online resource aimed at delivering high-quality up-to-date information about skin diseases to health care consumers. The Web site was started in 2006 and has since earned several awards in the category of consumer health care Web sites. The authors of the site are physicians, with most being board-certified dermatologists. The Chair of the Editorial Board is Dr. Lowell Goldsmith, an accomplished academic dermatologist who has served as Editor-in-Chief of the *Journal of Investigative Dermatology* for many years. The Web site was developed by Logical Images, a private company based in Rochester, New York. Logical Images is the parent company for Visual Dx Health and Visual Dx, the powerful subscription version for clinicians that has more detailed information on diagnosis and treatment. Funding for the Web site comes from third-party advertisements.

The quality of health care information varies widely, and the recommendation of trustworthy Web sites would help our patients in their pursuit of information.[17] Visual Dx Health users can find information on a skin disease by browsing through an alphabetic list of more than 170 diagnoses. Alternatively, users can generate a differential diagnosis by entering age, gender, and body location. After a user selects a diagnosis, a general overview of the disease is given, along with images and references. The printer-friendly option makes this Web site a great supplemental resource for physicians when patients desire more information about their diagnoses. Additionally, Visual Dx Health users can perform a Google-powered "VisualDx trusted search," which attempts to weed out some of the low-quality Web sites and provides a list of links that have been approved and deemed trustworthy by the Editorial Board.

Medical school curricula increasingly use online teaching resources. Online resources are a valuable aspect of undergraduate medical education as medical school class sizes grow and the number of academic dermatologists struggles to keep up.[18,19] Learning dermatology is particularly amenable to a computer-based program with high-quality images, because dermatology is a field that relies largely on pattern recognition.[20] Various educational tools and applications on the (Logical Images) Web site are useful for teaching fundamental dermatologic principles to medical students and residents. Several free interactive lessons with quizzes focus on morphology, the basic skin examination, and pattern recognition.

Table 1
Clinical resources for dermatologists that include web sites with image databases and freely accessible peer-reviewed research

Web Site	Web Site Address	Funding	Comments
Select open access dermatology journals: *BMC Dermatology* *The Open Dermatology Journal*	http://www.biomedcentral.com/bmcdermatol/ http://www.bentham.org/open/todj/	Author fees	Offers free online access to all articles.
National Library of Health Skin Disorder Specialist Library	http://www.library.nhs.uk/skin	National Health Service National Library for Health	Offers an up-to-date collection of reviewed evidence and documents on skin conditions. Free links to guidelines for treatment and has patient information resources
New Zealand Dermatologic Society, Incorporated	http://www.dermnet.org.nz/	Various industry sponsors	Web site provides diagnostic information, pictures, and treatments for common and rare dermatologic diseases. Web site also features quizzes and online courses.
Johns Hopkins point of case information technology ABX guide	http://prod.hopkins-abxguide.org/	Currently sponsored by Schering-Plough (corporation does not have input regarding Web site content)	User selects from a list of common infectious dermatologic diagnoses. Web site gives information about the pathogen, clinical manifestations, and various antibiotic treatment regimens.
Medline Plus for skin and nails	http://www.nlm.nih.gov/medlineplus/skinhairandnails.html	US National Library of Medicine and the National Institutes of Health	User can select from a list of common dermatologic diagnoses or can search based on whether there is hair, skin, or nail involvement. Web site gives links to overviews, recent research (abstracts and references), and current clinical trials.
Global skin atlas	http://www.globalskinatlas.com/index.cfm Sister Web sites: http://www.dermoscopyatlas.com/ http://www.globalskinpathatlas.com/	Privately funded and maintained	Users can search photographs of 798 rare and common dermatologic diseases. Web site also features a quiz. Sister Web sites include the dermoscopy atlas and the global skin path atlas.

Abbreviation: ABX, antibiotics.

Table 2
Web sites with dermatology-related educational materials for patients, medical students, and residents

Web Site	Web Site Address	Funding	Comments
Map of dermatology	http://healthcybermap.org/dermap/	Privately funded and maintained	This Google images interface allows users to enter body region and morphology to generate a brief differential. After selecting diagnosis, a Google search generates images.
Virtual grand rounds in dermatology 2.0	http://vgrd.blogspot.com/ (web 2.0 version) www.vgrd.org	Privately funded and maintained	Difficult cases are presented, and viewers are given the opportunity to comment and evaluate by means of an open Web 2.0 platform. Faculty members from around the world are listed, and membership from developing nations is encouraged.
Visual Dx Health Logical Images	http://www.visualdxhealth.com/ http://www.logicalimages.com/ educationalTools/learnDerm.htm	Various industry sponsors	Web site provides information on 10 common skin conditions. One can also search for diagnoses by selecting body area affected, gender, and patient age. An excellent patient education resource.
Derm Help Central	http://dermatologycentral.typepad.com/resource/	Privately funded and maintained	This Web site provides synopses and links to the latest patient-directed dermatology news articles. It also posts PDF files with helpful information, such as dry skin care, how to apply Aldara, and examples of a brisk reaction.

Table 3
Evidence-based medicine resources for dermatologists that promote literature appraisal and collaboration

Web Site	Web Site Address	Funding	Comments
JournalReview.org	www.journalreview.org	Privately owned company	This Web site is an online journal club, where users can read and contribute to discussions about medical literature.
ebderm.org	www.ebderm.org	Created in conjunction with Center for Evidence-Based Dermatology, grant from Sulzberger Institute	Web site offers resources for performing literature searches, guide to web-based resources, library of materials, and online forum.
Cochrane Skin Group	http://www.csg.cochrane.org/en/index.html	Affiliated with the Center for Evidence-Based Dermatology, received grant from National Institute for Health Research	An expert panel reviews published and unpublished evidence to answer clinical questions and offer evidence-based recommendations. Free access to abstracts and summaries.
Center for Evidence-Based Dermatology	http://www.nottingham.ac.uk/dermatology/	Funding provided by the UK Department of Health's National Institute for Health Research	Web site lists references of peer-reviewed publications related to the center's research. The major clinical research focus is atopic dermatitis. Offers eczema diagnostic tools and outcome measures.

Visual Dx Health and the Logical Images Web sites provide high-quality information, educational materials, and images with applications appropriate for patients and medical trainees.

EVIDENCE BASED MEDICINE: WWW.JOURNALREVIEW.ORG

Many physicians belong to a journal club, where they meet to discuss medical literature and begin to translate evidence-based medicine into personal practice. Time invested in journal clubs is viewed by most physicians as well spent, likely because preparing and discussing the literature is an active learning process. In one study, residents and faculty placed higher educational value on journal clubs than on grand rounds or didactic lectures.[21] The Web site JournalReview.org is designed as an online journal club and is meant to complement the practice of traditional journal clubs. One benefit of the online journal club is that clinicians can read the literature and participate at their leisure. With an online resource, the clinician's time can be more wisely spent in practicing critical appraisal skills and asking questions pertinent to his or her personal practice.[22] The Web site is currently owned by a privately held firm whose founders envisioned it serving as an international Internet-based forum for clinicians to review and discuss medical literature. The site's business plan anticipates increasing collaboration with commercial Internet content providers to provide long-term sustainability.

JournalReview.org is a user-friendly Web site with a variety of links for searching and appraising medical literature. After entering a keyword, the Web site performs a PubMed query in search of journal articles and delivers a list of references with links to abstracts. One can also search for recently discussed articles and peruse dialog contributed by members by following links to different medical specialties. After completing the fast and free registration process, one can participate in the online forum. Users of the site can sign up for live Really Simple Syndication (RSS) feeds for a particular journal club or specialty so that they can be updated when new comments are added to a given forum.[23] Common ways to contribute to the forum include posing questions, sharing appraisals or criticisms of the evidence, or summarizing the discussion generated by a group in a traditional journal club. When an article stimulates dialog among different users, the Web site sends an automatic notification to the author of the paper as well as to other experts in the field, further enriching discussion of the topic at hand.

As public servants, physicians have the responsibility to interpret and evaluate new scientific research. Pharmaceutical representatives frequently visit doctor's offices and present impressive statistics showing that their expensive patented drugs are superior to the alternatives. Often, funding for the studies cited by the representatives comes from drug companies looking to profit. The data are construed to show the marketed drug in the most favorable light, with useful information (eg, a cost-benefit analysis with similar generic medications) often omitted. JournalReview.org provides a forum where clinicians can discuss the literature in a transparent way. This decreases bias and enables the medical community to identify the true value of a study for themselves.

As the use of this resource increases, creators of the Web site are eager to modify and improve it to facilitate interpretation and discussion of the literature further. The Medical Society of the State of New York (MSSNY) has recently partnered with JournalReview.org to create an online journal club for their members. The popularity of scientific interest groups on social networking sites, such as Facebook.com, has been growing, likely because it is convenient to participate in social and professional networking at the same time.[24] Facebook use is common among medical trainees, with 44.5% of medical students and residents having accounts with the Web site.[25] In an effort to reach out to the next generation of clinicians, Journal Review.org has recently partnered with Facebook, and the interface allows users to stay in touch with colleagues by discussing medical literature.

In conclusion, JournalReview.org is an excellent free tool for clinicians around the world who strive to keep up to date with evidence-based medicine by critically appraising the latest medical literature.

SUMMARY

Many Internet resources for dermatologists benefit public health by providing education and information on the diagnosis and treatment of skin conditions. A variety of dermatology resources exist on the Web, but finding quality resources can be time-consuming. The authors provide a collection of high-quality, freely accessible, English-language Web sites that they have categorized as clinical, educational, or evidence-based medicine resources. They hope that this list of sources helps to meet the informational needs of dermatologists and promotes awareness and education on skin diseases.

REFERENCES

1. Open access day—October 14, 2008: about the movement. Available at: http://openaccessday.org/what-is-open-access/. Accessed January 8, 2009.
2. Jacobson CC, Resneck JS Jr, Kimball AB. Generational differences in practice patterns of dermatologists in the United States: implications for workforce planning. Arch Dermatol 2004;140:1477–82.
3. Davies K. The information-seeking behaviour of doctors: a review of the evidence. Health Info Libr J 2007;24:78–94.
4. Tang H, Ng JH. Googling for a diagnosis—use of Google as a diagnostic aid: Internet based study. BMJ 2006;333:1143–5.
5. Grindlay D, Boulos MN, Williams HC. Introducing the national library for health skin conditions specialist library. BMC Dermatol 2005;5:4.
6. Papadavid E, Falagas ME. World Wide Web resources of open access, educational dermatology clinical image quizzes and databases. J Am Acad Dermatol 2007;56:e81–5.
7. Huang ST, Kamel Boulos MN, Dellavalle RP. Scientific discourse 2.0. Will your next poster session be in second life? EMBO Rep 2008;9:496–9.
8. McGee JB, Begg M. What medical educators need to know about "Web 2.0". Med Teach 2008;30:164–9.
9. Johnson KR, Freeman SR, Dellavalle RP. Wikis: the application of Web 2.0. Arch Dermatol 2007;143:1065–6.
10. Giustini D. How Web 2.0 is changing medicine. BMJ 2006;333:1283–4.
11. Gonzalez-Gonzalez AI, Dawes M, Sanchez-Mateos J, et al. Information needs and information-seeking behavior of primary care physicians. Ann Fam Med 2007;5:345–52.
12. Godlee F. Open access to research. BMJ 2008;337:a1051.
13. National Institute of Health. Public access homepage. Available at: http://publicaccess.nih.gov/. Accessed January 8, 2009.
14. Dellavalle RP, Banks MA, Ellis JI. Self-archiving dermatology articles. J Am Acad Dermatol 2008;59:1086–8.
15. Hesse BW, Nelson DE, Kreps GL, et al. Trust and sources of health information: the impact of the Internet and its implications for health care providers: findings from the first health information national trends survey. Arch Intern Med 2005;165:2618–24.
16. Tu HT, Cohen GR. Striking jump in consumers seeking health care information. Track Rep 2008;20:1–8.
17. Dutta-Bergman M. Trusted online sources of health information: differences in demographics, health beliefs, and health-information orientation. J Med Internet Res 2003;5(3):e21.
18. Loo DS, Liu CL, Geller AC, et al. Academic dermatology manpower: issues of recruitment and retention. Arch Dermatol 2007;143:341–7.
19. Farrimond H, Dornan TL, Cockcroft A, et al. Development and evaluation of an e-learning package for teaching skin examination. Action research. Br J Dermatol 2006;155:592–9.
20. Jenkins S, Goel R, Morrell DS. Computer-assisted instruction versus traditional lecture for medical student teaching of dermatology morphology: a randomized control trial. J Am Acad Dermatol 2008;59:255–9.
21. Elnicki DM, Halperin AK, Shockcor WT, et al. Multidisciplinary evidence-based medicine journal clubs: curriculum design and participants' reactions. Am J Med Sci 1999;317:243–6.
22. Doust J, Del Mar CB, Montgomery BD, et al. EBM journal clubs in general practice. Aust Fam Physician 2008;37:54–6.
23. Ward JA. RSS feeds: sweating the really simple stuff. Toxicol Pathol 2007;35:846–7.
24. Bailey DS, Zanders ED. Drug discovery in the era of Facebook—new tools for scientific networking. Drug Discov Today 2008;13:863–8.
25. Thompson LA, Dawson K, Ferdig R, et al. The intersection of online social networking with medical professionalism. J Gen Intern Med 2008;23:954–7.

Reviewing Dermatology Manuscripts and Publications

Christina A. Nelson, MD[a], Scott R. Freeman, MD[b],
Robert P. Dellavalle, MD, PhD, MSPH[b,c,d],*

KEYWORDS

- Manuscript • Peer review • Epidemiology
- Public health • Dermatology

Why do authors write? Simply put, they write to convey a message. The type and standards of writing are determined by what message the author would like to convey and who the audience is. Scientific writing in particular is held to rigorous standards to ensure quality and accuracy of the message. One of the most important aspects of these standards is peer review, in which submitted work is reviewed by experts in the field who ideally provide constructive feedback.

Peer review is vital to the quality of scientific publications;[1,2] however, physicians and scientists receive little formal training on how to review a manuscript.[3,4] Guidelines on manuscript review are occasionally published in the scientific literature,[5,6] but they are often specialty-specific and little has been published in the dermatologic literature.

The importance of public health has become increasingly apparent in the medical field and specifically in dermatology. Sun safety, prevention of allergic skin disorders, etiology and management of psoriasis, and many other dermatologic disorders have all been guided by epidemiologic research and have significant public health implications. Epidemiologic studies can and will continue to contribute a great deal to the dermatologic

literature. Accordingly, it is essential for reviewers to be familiar with the guidelines for epidemiologic research to uphold the scientific rigor of published studies.

Postpublication review is becoming increasingly popular in the Internet era, making it possible for any reader to act as a reviewer. One such example is the British Medical Journal's "rapid responses" feature,[7] which allows readers to post electronic letters to the editor that can be viewed online alongside the original article. Journalreview.org[8] compiles and lists post-publication reviews from a variety of journals by specialty. This article may also serve as a useful guideline when writing post-publication reviews and critiques.

REVIEWING PRINCIPLES

Performing a relevant literature search and critiquing a manuscript takes time, and most journals request a response within 14 days.[9] It is imperative that both authors and journals receive reviews in a timely fashion, since a delay on the reviewer's part can significantly inhibit the publication process. Decline an invitation to review if you have inadequate time to perform the review.

The authors thank Allan Prochazka, MD, MSc for comments on the manuscript.
We had no source of funding, nor conflicts of interest to declare.
[a] Department of Preventive Medicine and Biometrics, University of Colorado at Denver, Building 500, Box B119, 13001 E 17th Place, Aurora, CO 80045, USA
[b] Department of Dermatology, University of Colorado Denver, School of Medicine, P.O. Box 6510, Mail Stop F703, Aurora, CO 80045-6510, USA
[c] Department of Veterans Affairs Medical Center, 1055 Clermont Street #165, Denver, CO 80220, USA
[d] Colorado School of Public Health, 13001 E. 17th Place, Campus Box B119, Aurora, CO, 80045, USA
* Corresponding author. Colorado School of Public Health, 13001 E. 17th Place, Campus Box B119, Aurora, CO, 80045.
E-mail address: robert.dellavalle@ucdenver.edu (R.P. Dellavalle).

Dermatol Clin 27 (2009) 201–204
doi:10.1016/j.det.2008.11.005

Respect those involved in the review process. Review as you would want your work to be reviewed; provide constructive comments. Be fair and remember that the final decision rests with the editor.

Do not review studies if you possess a potential conflict of interest with the work.[10] Also, be sure to maintain confidentiality of the authors and the study if indicated.[11]

INITIAL REVIEW

Take a quick read and note anything you love, hate, or don't understand. Note your overall gut feeling. Does the study advance useful knowledge in the field? Are all of the necessary parts of the abstract, text, and references present and in the proper form? What kind of paper is it? Are there any serious flaws in the design, and if so can they be repaired?

Decide if the paper aligns with the journal's aim and scope, and whether it will appeal to readers. Familiarize yourself with the journal's instructions to authors. If the authors have failed to follow the journal's instructions to authors, make notations regarding what should be corrected. If there are flagrant violations of the requirements, send the manuscript back to the editor and request that the authors properly revise the manuscript to conform to journal requirements before proceeding.

If the manuscript is in order, read it again carefully and begin the review. Number the comments and indicate the location in the manuscript to which they pertain. List problems clearly and succinctly, and provide references for your statements when possible.

TITLE PAGE

The title should be informative, succinct, and accurate. The main purpose is to relay the bottom line results clearly. If you can think of a better title, suggest it.

In addition, the title page should

- specifically state the design (case study, randomized control trial, systematic review, etc.);
- include appropriate keywords;
- list all authors with their affiliations (and highest educational degrees if required by the journal);
- cite funding sources and conflicts of interest.

ABSTRACT

Many online researchers view only an abstract, therefore it must suffice on its own to convey the paper's message clearly. The results section of the abstract should include the most important numerical results from the study. As you are reviewing the paper, make sure the conclusions presented in the abstract are supported by the study's data.

INTRODUCTION

The introduction should be brief, so point out any non-essential paragraphs, sentences or words. It should clearly state the problem and relevance, hypothesis, and objectives of the study. Review information should be limited but supported by textbook or other review material; references should point readers outside the field to other useful resources.

METHODS: QUALITY GUIDELINES FOR EPIDEMIOLOGIC STUDIES

The methods section is the heart of any paper and often the most poorly written. It should delineate the study setting, population, recruitment, design, and statistical analysis. The methods must contain sufficient details to repeat the work. If not, what additional information is needed? In addition, it is often helpful for the authors to describe how they reviewed the literature in preparation for their work.

The STROBE statement (Strengthening the Reporting of Observational Studies in Epidemiology) was published in 2007 to provide guidelines on how to report observational research clearly and accurately.[12] These recommendations include cross-sectional, case-control, and cohort study designs and were developed to improve transparency, accuracy, and generalizability of observational study publications. Reviewers should be familiar with the STROBE statement and incorporate its recommendations into the assessment of an epidemiologic manuscript.

The CONSORT (Consolidated Standards of Reporting Trials) checklist and patient flow diagram are similar guidelines for randomized controlled trials (RCTs). They should be included in all RCT manuscripts and are available on the CONSORT Web site[13] and in other recent publications.[14,15]

The QUOROM (Quality of Reporting of Meta-analyses) statement provides a checklist of standards to improve the quality of reports of meta-analyses of RCTs.[16] There is also a flow diagram for studies to provide information about how RCTs were identified, included, and excluded, and the reasons for doing so.

A statement regarding review and approval by the appropriate human ethics committee is appropriate for research involving human subjects, and it should include the procedures used to obtain informed consent. If photographs are included, check that the authors have appropriate consent and have taken sufficient precautions to maintain confidentiality.[17]

RESULTS

The results should be a neutral description of the study findings; interpretation is saved for the discussion. The data should be presented clearly and concisely; tables and figures present results more efficiently than text. Duplicate presentation in both text and tables should be avoided. Make sure that each table, figure, and picture is essential; if any can be combined or reformatted, suggest they do so. Also check that the numbers in the tables are consistent and account for all of the data.

DISCUSSION

The discussion is a structured and succinct interpretation of the study results.[18] Do conclusions follow soundly from the results of the study? Are smaller, post hoc results given enormous thrust in this section while less flashy, primary data are largely ignored? The discussion should also comment on study relevance to the current body of literature, generalizability of findings, biases, and limitations.[19]

REFERENCES

Check that the most relevant and recent references are present. Are others needed? Confirm that reference articles actually are what they were referenced as; also check that all cited Web sites (Uniform Resource Locators [URLs]) are active.[20] Familiarize yourself with what the authors have published recently; all closely related papers written by the authors should be made available to assure that duplicate publication is not occurring.

ONLINE APPENDIX

If the journal allows online supplements, should any data be moved online? The reviewer may also suggest additional data or supplementary material that would be helpful to include online.[21,22] A podcast (an audio or video file) may greatly improve communication with the audience.

DETECTING PLAGIARISM AND DUPLICATE PUBLICATIONS

Recent editoral articles have highlighted the problem of plagiarism and duplicate publications in the scientific literature. There are several anti-plagiarism computer programs designed to identify such duplications—examples of commonly used programs include eTBlast, a free text-similarity based search engine,[23] and subscription-based CrossCheck[24] and Turnitin.[25] It is generally not the responsibility of the reviewer to apply these programs, however he or she should be aware of them.

FINAL THOUGHTS

Once you have finished the step-by-step review, write a brief summary of your thoughts to the editors. No need to introduce the review with a lengthy synopsis—a few sentences will do. Your comments on the manuscript will show that you have spent time digesting the paper.

Most journals receive a large volume of submissions and can only choose a limited number for publication. Your input on uniqueness of the study population, novel methods, and new approaches to diagnosis and treatment will assist editors with the decision to publish. If the paper is a new review, determine whether there has been an advance in the field that merits a new review.

Finally, the reviewer should make a recommendation to: accept, accept with minor revision, accept with major revision, or reject the manuscript. Include your rationale for the decision along with specific feedback on how to improve the paper.

REVIEWING REVISED MANUSCRIPTS

Once the review process has begun, changes to the text should be clearly marked with underlining or other means. Make sure that the authors have clearly addressed all previous comments. Avoid suggesting minor new changes or flip-flopping on a position taken in the primary review. New substantial issues may arise throughout the review process and should be addressed as needed.

CONCLUSION—THE REVIEWER'S TASK

Keep in mind that the ultimate purpose of reviewing manuscripts is to produce better publications and journals. Traditional peer review is vital to the publication of high quality peer-reviewed literature; additionally, in the Internet era postpublication review is increasingly important and allows every reader to become a reviewer. The time and effort you spend reviewing will be greatly appreciated as an important contribution to the field of medicine.

REFERENCES

1. Goodman SN, Berlin J, Fletcher SW, et al. Manuscript quality before and after peer review and editing at Annals of Internal Medicine. Ann Intern Med 1994;121:11–21.
2. Isohanni M. Peer review–still the well-functioning quality control and enhancer in scientific research. Acta Psychiatr Scand 2005;112:165–6.
3. Snell L, Spencer J. Reviewers' perceptions of the peer review process for a medical education journal. Med Educ 2005;39(1):90–7.
4. Benos DJ, Kirk KL, Hall JE. How to review a paper. Adv Physiol Educ 2003;27:47–52.
5. Bourne P, Korngreen A. Ten simple rules for reviewers. PLoS Comput Biol 2006;2(9):e110.
6. Hoppin F. How I review an original scientific article. Am J Respir Crit Care Med 2002;166(8):1019–23.
7. BMJ rapid responses. Available at: http://resources.bmj.com/bmj/readers/responding-to-articles. Accessed November 4, 2008.
8. Journal review. Available at: http://journalreview.org. Accessed November 4, 2008.
9. Noseworthy J, Gross R, Engel A. Message from the editors to our US and international reviewers. Neurology 2008;70:92–96.
10. Bland C, Caelleigh A, Steinecke A. Reviewer's etiquette. Acad Med 2001;76(9):954–5.
11. Dellavalle RP. Cultivating peer review. J Am Acad Dermatol 2006;55:1113–5.
12. von Elm E, Altman DG, Egger M, et al. The Strengthening the Reporting of Observational Studies in Epidemiology (STROBE) statement: guidelines for reporting observational studies. PLoS Med 2007;4(10):e296.
13. CONSORT statement Web site. Available at: http://www.consort-statement.org. Accessed November 4, 2008.
14. Hopewell S, Clarke M, Moher D, et al. CONSORT Group. CONSORT for reporting randomized controlled trials in journal and conference abstracts: explanation and elaboration. PLoS Med 2008;5(1):e20.
15. Piaggio G, Elbourne DR, Altman DG, et al. CONSORT Group. Reporting of noninferiority and equivalence randomized trials: an extension of the CONSORT statement. JAMA 2006;295(10):1152–60.
16. Moher D, Cook DJ, Eastwood S, et al. Improving the quality of reports of meta-analyses of randomised controlled trials: the QUOROM statement. Lancet 1999;354(9193):1896–900.
17. Scheinfeld N. Photographic images, digital imaging, dermatology, and the law. Arch Dermatol 2004;140(4):473–6.
18. Docherty M, Smith R. The case for structuring the discussion of scientific papers. BMJ 1999;318(7193):1224–5.
19. Dellavalle RP. Limitations. J Am Acad Dermatol 2004;51:678.
20. Dellavalle RP, Hester EJ, Heilig LF, et al. Going, going, gone: the loss of internet references in medical and scientific publications. Science 2003;302:787–8.
21. Dellavalle RP, Lundahl K, Freeman SR, et al. Journals should set a new standard in transparency. Nature 2007;445:364.
22. Freeman SR, Lundahl K, Schilling LM, et al. Human research review committee requirements in medical journals. Clin Invest Med 2008;31(1):E49–54.
23. eTBLAST. Available at: http://invention.swmed.edu/etblast/index.shtml. Accessed November 4, 2008.
24. Crosscheck. Available at: http://www.crossref.org. Accessed November 4, 2008.
25. Turnitin. Available at: http://turnitin.com. Accessed November 4, 2008.

Melanoma Epidemiology and Public Health

Marianne Berwick, PhD, MPH[a,b,*], Esther Erdei, PhD[a],
Jennifer Hay, PhD[c]

KEYWORDS

- Melanoma • Mortality • Incidence

Melanoma has presented a conundrum to physicians and prevention researchers. We should be able to reduce incidence and mortality rather easily because evolving melanoma lesions are observable on the surface of the skin. However, melanoma has not proved tractable. The incidence and mortality have risen in all developed countries during the past 50 years. However, mortality appears to be abating among younger cohorts even though the reason for this is not clear.

EPIDEMIOLOGY

The epidemiology of melanoma is marked by contrasts. The majority of melanomas are diagnosed at very thin (<1 mm Breslow thickness) and highly curable stages—about 70 percent in most series. However, melanomas diagnosed later (those with Breslow thickness >1 mm) have much poorer survival rates and there are no satisfactory cures for advanced melanoma.

Furthermore, melanoma is more often diagnosed among advantaged individuals within a population, but the disadvantaged individuals are more likely to have advanced disease.[1–3] Whether this is due to host factors associated with deprivation, such as life stress, or to factors associated with access to care, such as distance to providers, is not well understood. Finally, cutaneous melanoma is most common among developed countries with large numbers of white residents, while it is rare and presents with different phenotype and histology in less developed countries and in other ethnic groups. Current estimates place the number of new cases of melanoma at 160,177 worldwide and deaths from melanoma at 40,781.[4] In the United States, there were an estimated 62,480 new cases of melanoma diagnosed in 2008, and 8420 deaths from melanoma.[5] Although the number of new cases appears to be increasing, the mortality rates appear to be decreasing among younger cohorts of melanoma patients.[6] In addition, some of the incidence increase is certainly artifactual as we are certainly looking harder for melanoma as evidenced by the increasing rates of biopsy, and we are finding lesions today that 20 years ago would never have been called melanoma.[7,8] In the meantime, scientists cannot differentiate melanomas that will progress from those that are indolent; therefore, it is imperative that research continues to investigate the best means for prevention.

Risk Factors

Risk factors for melanoma can generally be divided into environmental and genetic. The search to understand the interaction of the two has been facilitated by advances in genomics.

This work was supported by Grant CA112524 from the National Cancer Institute.

[a] Division of Epidemiology and Biostatistics, Department of Internal Medicine, 1 University of New Mexico, MSC08 4360, CRF 103A, Albuquerque, NM 87131 0001, USA

[b] Population Science, University of New Mexico Cancer Center, Albuquerque, NM 87131, USA

[c] Department of Psychiatry and Behavioral Sciences, Memorial Sloan-Kettering Cancer Center, 641 Lexington Avenue, 7th Floor, New York, NY 10022, USA

* Corresponding author. Division of Epidemiology, MSC08 4360, CRF 103A, 1 University of New Mexico, Albuquerque, NM 87131 0001.

E-mail address: mberwick@salud.unm.edu (M. Berwick).

derm.theclinics.com

Environmental risk factors

Sunlight Ultraviolet radiation (UVR) is the major known etiologic agent associated with melanoma. Many individuals however do not know that different patterns of sun exposure have different effects in the development of melanoma. For example, chronic sun exposure, that which one receives during outdoor work on a daily basis, does not increase risk for melanoma and is even associated with inhibition of melanoma.[9–11] On the other hand, intermittent sun exposure, large blasts of UVR, received on weekends or holidays, is the major form of UVR promoting the development of melanoma.[12]

Measurement of intermittent sun exposure or recreational sun exposure represents an important research challenge because measures of past sun exposure necessarily depend on subject recall of exposure, which is not always reliable.[13] Epidemiologic studies have shown weak associations between episodes of sunburn and melanoma incidence.[14] Estimates of the effect of intermittent exposure have ranged from a protective effect of (a relative risk) of 0.44 (0.21–0.91)[15] to an adverse risk of 8.41 (3.63–19.6).[16] Imprecise measurement associated with self-reports is an important rate-limiting factor in determining the relationship between intermittent sun exposure and melanoma incidence.

Furthermore, excessive sunlight exposure in youth, among individuals with aberrant nevogenesis, increases the risk of melanoma, particularly for melanoma associated with BRAF mutations;[17,18] whereas continuous, intermittent sun exposure over a lifetime, are associated with NRAS mutations among older individuals.

Other sources of ultraviolet radiation Mounting evidence points to the negative effects of tanning beds.[19] In 2006, the International Agency for Research on Cancer convened an expert panel of epidemiologists to evaluate the risks for melanoma and other skin cancers from use of sunbeds.[20] They performed a meta-analysis of 19 studies that have evaluated the association between sunbed exposure and melanoma and other skin cancers. The study showed that early life exposure is the most damaging. In this meta-analysis the relative risk for melanoma was 1.75 (95% confidence interval [CI],1.35–2.26) for "first exposure under the age of 35;" a relative risk of 1.15 that is statistically significant (95% CI, 1.00–1.31) for "ever use;" a summary relative risk of 1.49 (95% CI, 0.93–2.38) for exposure distant in time; and a summary relative risk of 1.10 (95% CI, 0.76–1.60) for recent exposure. All of the relative risks are higher than 1.0. The most persuasive

study a (prospective cohort study of 106,379 women in Sweden and Norway) found, not only a similar level of risk, but that the increased risk was not due to the type of UV lamps used before 1983 but likely due to more recent types of sunbeds.[21]

Host factors

Melanocytic nevi Nevi are the strongest risk factor for the development of melanoma. Studies have shown that those with a higher than average number of moles (often counted on the back, and 40 or more on the back can be considered high). The way in which nevi might be involved in risk has been considered in different ways. One theory is that nevi are actually on the causal pathway, and that some nevi develop into melanoma. This theory is supported by the approximately 40% of melanomas that have an adjacent nevus or nevus remnant still observable by pathology.[22,23]

Individuals with fewer nevi require repeated exposure to sunlight to drive carcinogenesis because they are more likely to develop melanomas on high sun exposure areas such as the head and neck, while those with many nevi, who are more likely to develop melanoma of the trunk, may possess host factors that drive carcinogenesis after minimal sunlight exposure.[18] Therefore, it is plausible that the oncogenic pathway characterized by pigment cell instability is associated with a higher number of nevi and may lead to more aggressive melanoma and a worse prognosis.

In any case, having more nevi than average, or having dysplastic nevi, increases risk for melanoma substantially.[24–26]

Family history First-degree relatives of melanoma patients have a higher risk of the disease than individuals without positive family history, suggesting that a distinct hereditary component exists. Familial melanoma accounts for an estimated 5 to 10 percent of all cases of melanoma.[27] Characteristics which distinguish the familial from the nonfamilial form of the disease include younger age at first diagnosis, better survival, thinner lesions, multiple primary lesions, and increased occurrence of nonmelanoma cancers.[28] Pooled data from eight case-control studies showed that an individual's risk of melanoma increases by about twofold with an affected first-degree relative.[29] This effect was independent of host factors such as age, nevus count, hair and eye color, and freckling. Familial relative risk remained similar in all of the studies, even though melanoma incidence varied by about 10-fold in the study areas.

Phenotypic characteristics Phenotype is independently important as a risk factor for the development of melanoma: light hair color, light eye color, and light skin color, including skin that freckles easily. These phenotypic characteristics are often subsumed under the heading of "skin type." Fitzpatrick[30] classified skin type into six groups that are frequently used even though the reproducibility of these groupings is relatively poor (Table 1).[31]

Variation in susceptibility genes
Major advances in genetics have made it possible to identify genetic factors that are critical to susceptibility to melanoma. The Genome Wide Association Studies (GWAS) have identified new variants in genes that may be found to play an important role in the development of melanoma.

Pigmentation genes Foremost among the pigmentary genes known to be associated with melanoma is the melanocortin 1 receptor (MC1R). Data show that some MC1R variants are associated both with melanoma and phenotype—particularly red hair. Others are only associated with melanoma development, suggesting that MC1R variants could play a role in melanoma development by way of pigmentary and nonpigmentary pathways.[32] Pigmentary and other genes have recently been identified by GWAS, and their effects remain to be evaluated.[33,34]

DNA repair genes Genetic variants in DNA repair genes are obvious candidates for melanoma susceptibility based on the xeroderma pigmentosum (XP) paradigm.[35] XP patients have an approximately 1,000-fold increased risk for developing melanoma and variants of XP, and other repair genes have recently been associated with risk.[36,37]

Cell cycle genes To date, few mutations have been found in cell cycle genes in melanoma etiology.[38,39] The familial melanoma gene, CDKN2A, is rarely mutated among those with sporadic melanoma, although it accounts for approximately 30 percent of mutations in those with a hereditary form of the disease.[40]

Gene–environment interaction
The pattern of sun exposure that appears to induce skin cancer, in particular melanoma, development is complex and is clearly different by skin type (ie, propensity to burn, ability to tan). Armstrong and colleagues[41] have proposed a model consistent with data from other epidemiologic studies where risk for melanoma increases with increasing sun exposure among those who tan easily, but only with a small amount after which risk decreases with increasing exposure. Among subjects who are intermediate in their ability to tan, risk continues to increase slowly and then, at some point, declines with increasing exposure. On the other hand, those subjects who have great difficulty tanning have an almost linear increase in risk with increasing sun exposure. This model recognizes that individuals are differentially susceptible to sun exposure and have different levels of risk based on skin type. Moreover, it suggests that different types or patterns of sun exposure are associated with different levels of risk for melanoma.

PUBLIC HEALTH

Unfortunately, there is little sound evidence on which to move forward in public education and awareness of skin cancer. This is a critical juncture for the development of such evidence. Currently, different factions promulgate somewhat confusing recommendations: some advise avoiding the sun,

Table 1
Fitzpatrick classification of skin type

Skin Type	Skin Color	Characteristics
I	White, very fair, red or blond hair, blue eyes, freckles	Always burns, never tans
II	White; fair; red or blond hair; blue, hazel, or green eyes	Usually burns, tans with difficulty
III	Cream white, fair with any eye or hair color, very common	Sometimes mild burn, gradually tans
IV	Brown, typical Mediterranean Caucasian skin	Rarely burns, tans with ease
V	Dark Brown, Mid-Eastern skin types	very rarely burns, tans very easily
VI	Black	Never burns, tans very easily

From Fitzpatrick TB. The validity and practicality of sun-reactive skin types I through VI. 1988; Arch Dermatol 124:869–71; with permission.

and others advise enjoying a moderate amount of sun exposure. The tanning industry is even promoting the use of tanning parlors to develop a "safe" tan.

The American Cancer Society[42] recommends sun protection strategies including sun avoidance between 10 AM and 4 PM and, when sun cannot be avoided, use of umbrellas, protective hats, clothing, and sunscreen with a sun protection factor of 15 or more. Total avoidance of artificial UV sources such as tanning beds is also recommended. Unfortunately, less than half (47%) of the United States population engages in any sun protection,[43] and 59% report that they have sunbathed in the past year.[44] Data from over 28,000 individuals in the 2005 National Health Interview Survey[45] showed that only about half (43%–51% across age groups) reported frequent (sometimes/most of the time/always) use of sunscreen, 65% to 80% did not usually stay in the shade when outside on a sunny day, and 15% to 51% used sun protection clothing. For each behavior, younger age was related to higher levels of risk behavior.

Educational Strategies

Programs for the general population

General population approaches to improve overall sun protection have been adopted most prominently in Australia. For example, the Australian state of Victoria adopted the SunSmart program integrating environmental change and mass media public education to address sun protection across the entire population. Documentation of this program shows that a mix of strategies is effective but quite expensive in improving sun protection behaviors.[46]

The "Slip, Slap, Slop" campaign has promoted sun protection for more than 20 years throughout Australia.[47] In Queensland, Australia, Stanton and colleagues[48] evaluated the effectiveness of one intensive campaign. They found that individuals did protect themselves when in the sun or, if they did not, they did not think they were out long enough to be sunburned. The motivation for protection stemmed from a desire to prevent future health problems, and it seems that the sun protective behaviors were a direct result of public health campaigns. However, they suggest that public health campaigns need to move beyond the current efforts to increase awareness and knowledge of skin cancer to provide supportive environments (shade is an issue in places like Australia and New Mexico) and enhance individual skills (such as recognition of the UV Index [UVI]).

Physician counseling

The Task Force on Community Preventive Services,[49] a Centers for Disease Control and Prevention group, has found adequate evidence to show that sun exposure is associated with the development of melanoma, but inadequate evidence to indicate that physician counseling will change patient behaviors to reduce risk.

Programs for high risk populations

Children In the United States, targeted approaches to specific higher-risk populations have been the predominant approach to intervention development. For example, interventions targeted to children are arguably quite important given that children spend a greater proportion of their time outdoors, and because sun exposure and sunburns (in particular before age 18) represent a large proportion of the lifetime environmental risk of skin cancer. Sun protection programs for children include interventions focused on parent behaviors, preschool children, and school-age children. Many of these interventions have been implemented in schools and hospitals. In general, those multiunit programs that occur over several sessions with intensive instruction work best.[50] However, widespread dissemination of these interventions may be limited by shrinking resources and competing demands in the school and other institutional environments.

Unfortunately, the Community Preventive Services Task Force[49] reported that education and policy approaches to increasing sun protective behaviors were effective when implemented in primary schools and in recreational or tourism settings, but found insufficient evidence to determine effectiveness when implemented in other settings, such as child care centers, secondary schools and colleges, and occupational settings. They also found "insufficient evidence to determine the effectiveness of interventions oriented to healthcare settings and providers, media campaigns alone, interventions oriented to parents or caregivers of children, and community-wide multicomponent interventions."

Family history of melanoma Another population that has been recently targeted for intervention has included those with a family history of melanoma, who face increased risks for skin cancer over and above the general population. For instance, Geller and colleagues[51] developed a novel telephone motivational interviewing and tailored education material approach, but the intervention did not show differential improvement in the treatment over the control group.

Interventions in high risk environments A final distinct intervention approach includes those interventions that are specific to various higher risk environments, and thus capitalize on the local situational cues in certain environments. For example, a program implemented at a zoo which included signage linking sun protection to animals' strategies of skin protection, tip sheets for parents, children's activities, and discounted sun protection was useful in increasing sales of sunscreen and hats compared with a control zoo.[52] Environmentally specific interventions have also been instituted at beaches, ski resorts, and swimming pools.[53–55]

The Use of Sunscreens

It is still not clear that sunscreens of any sort will provide protection from developing melanoma although they clearly prevent sunburn—a sign that sensitive skin has had too much UV. Suggestions have been made that sunscreens actually increase risk for skin cancer,[56] although the most likely way that this association might occur is when individuals use sunscreens to prolong their stay in the sun. Therefore, it is possible that the use of sunscreens for intentional sun exposure may actually increase risk. Sunscreen sun protection recommendations have been made by the International Agency for Research on Cancer.[57] No conclusion could be drawn about the cancer-preventive activity of topical use of sunscreens against basal-cell carcinoma and cutaneous melanoma. Unfortunately, based on data from carefully conducted studies, sunscreens are being used as tanning aids to avoid sunburn.[58]

The use of sunscreens has long been promoted as the first line of defense for prevention all types of skin cancer. However, during the last 10 years, the public has been warned not to rely on sunscreens alone, but to practice overall sun protection. Uncontrollable confounding limits the ability of an observational study to assess the efficacy of sunscreens. Therefore, individuals who are most at risk, those who are redheaded or a very light phenotype with poor tanning ability, or those who are planning to spend time at the beach after being in the office all day, are the ones who are most likely use sunscreens.

Since the 1990s, however, improvements have been made and sunscreens now cover a much broader portion of the UV spectrum.[59] We will be able to evaluate their effectiveness after a suitable lag period, such as 20 years, has passed.

A few randomized trials have evaluated the effects of sunscreens on a putative precursor lesion for melanoma, the development of nevi. Gallagher and colleagues[60] found a small effect of sunscreens in reducing nevus formation among those who freckled; the effect was extremely small

although statistically significant. Additionally, an observational study in Queensland, found that sun protection, including frequent reapplication of sunscreen, was associated with a reduced number of nevi in children between 1 and 3 years old.[61] In addition, van der Pols and colleagues[62] found that after participation in a trial of the use of sunscreens, those who had been randomized to daily use continued to use sunscreens. Thus, although the investigators limit the interpretation of their findings because of a 63% response to their follow up, intensive encouragement over multiple time periods with a simple message may be more effective than the multicomponent messages delivered by community sun protection campaigns. A German study, using multiple methods for intervention, found no evidence that education and sunscreen use would affect the development of nevi in 1,232 children 2 to 7 years old after a 3-year intervention.[63]

Clothing as Protection

The most consistent and robust protection from UVR in relationship to melanoma is the physical barrier provided by hats, long sleeves, and long pants. Clothing is an ideal protective agent against the sun and has been used for hundreds of years in sunny countries like India and Egypt where people tend to cover up to prevent excessive sun exposure with long sleeves, long pants, and hats or turbans.

The use of clothing appears to reduce the number of nevi formed. However, these studies are of young children who may eventually achieve their full nevus density later. An intervention to retard the development of nevi with clothing and sun protection was only moderately successful—more so among boys.[64] In an observational analysis of the same subjects in this randomized study, clothing and staying indoors were associated with a reduced number of nevi, but wearing sunscreen while unclothed was not.[65] Others found[66] that children who wore clothing had fewer nevi and those who used sunscreen had more.

The Controversy About Vitamin D and Sun Exposure

Some sun exposure produces vitamin D synthesis, improves seasonal affective disorder, may help lower blood pressure, may be inversely associated with the incidence and mortality from a number of cancers, and is the treatment for polymorphic light eruption. Excessive sun exposure, particularly the intermittent pattern, is responsible for much of cutaneous malignant melanoma. Overexposure to UVR can lead to sunburn, immunologic changes, precipitation and exacerbation of photosensitivity, accelerated skin aging and skin cancer. These important problems need to be addressed with effective education.

It has been hypothesized that, in some cases, even more sun may be beneficial. One explanation for the rise in melanoma incidence that takes into account the different effects of chronic (or daily) and intermittent sun exposure (the type office workers get on weekends and holidays at the beach) proposes that as people have replaced outdoor occupations with indoor ones, they have experienced more intermittent sun exposure.[67] The decrease in outdoor occupations, or chronic exposure which is actually protective for melanoma, could explain the increase in melanoma incidence in Canada.

Diffey[68] effectively argues that the population attains adequate vitamin D through recreational activities. He carefully points out that increasing solar exposure would lead to an increase in skin cancer. The point of the present discussion is that individuals should take care in the sun and, at the same time, realize that a small amount of sun exposure is not bad.

Confusion due to messages about vitamin D and sun exposure

Lately, the public has received confusing messages owing to the increasing recognition of the role of Vitamin D in protecting against many internal cancers as well as other diseases. In the United Kingdom, Hiom[69] worries that "a growing body of literature suggesting a cancer protective role for vitamin D and sun exposure presents further challenges for skin cancer prevention campaigns, no more so than when exaggerated claims for the health benefits of sunbathing make the media spotlight. The UK population tends to need little encouragement to make the most of sunshine, and this is especially true for the younger generation who most need to take care. Public health messages to avoid the midday sun, not to burn and to protect children should not adversely affect outdoor activity or population vitamin D levels, but it is important that they are targeted to those most at risk and are consistent." A number of groups—the Australian and New Zealand Bone and Mineral Society, Osteoporosis Australia, Australasian College of Dermatologists, the Cancer Council Australia, and others—have recently modified a long-standing message to the public from one of staying out of the sun to one of short periods of exposure for health.[70] Some argue in favor of "Love the sun and protect your skin" as a public health message.[71]

SOLUTIONS
The UV Index

The UVI is used in most developed countries and although many programs have been developed in the countries where light-skinned individuals predominate and also have high rates of skin cancer, the UVI is not used as widely as it might be.

The UVI should be studied more thoroughly to understand just how to best communicate levels of ground-level sun effects. Brooks and colleagues[72] have recently suggested that advocacy groups should work with the World Health Organization to lead such efforts. When comparing the promulgation of the UVI in three countries, the United States, the United Kingdom, and Australia, one sees widely differing presentation of the index, none of which appears to be effective as yet. As this is a widely-reported measure to assist individuals in enhancing their time outdoors, the New South Wales Cancer Council and the Anti-Cancer Council of Victoria[73] have suggested that it would be valuable to learn more about public perceptions of the index and how to enhance its use. Efforts should be made to seek media and other settings through which information concerning the UVI can be disseminated to reach population subgroups involved in activities and situations identified as at high risk for UV exposure. The groups suggest that priority be given to developing the following specific uses of the UVI:

- In daily weather forecasts to prompt appropriate sun protection behavior
- To improve understanding of the relationship between ambient temperature and ambient UV
- As a guide to seasonal changes in the times of and level of protection necessary during childhood outdoor activities, particularly in schools
- In sections of newspapers, magazines, radio programs and special cable TV channels aimed at high-risk groups or activities (eg, sports channels to target fishermen, cricketers, and sailors)
- In travel information targeted at Australian and international tourists.

Sun Exposure Behavior

The UVI can guide the need for protection. Sun exposure and sun protection are behaviorally controlled. It has recently been shown that the general population has a relatively accurate concept of skin cancer prevention.[50] However, high levels of knowledge about the risks of skin cancer do not necessarily translate into consistent sun protection. Indeed, this is the case for knowledge concerning diet and exercise recommendations as well, where knowledge is necessary but not sufficient to motivate behavior change.[74–76]

Given the prevailing belief that a suntan is attractive, concerns for appearance is a barrier to sun protection campaigns.[77] Accordingly, another important approach to promoting sun protection involves the use of appearance appeals, which are designed to emphasize the harm to physical appearance associated with sun exposure, or to increase the perceived attractiveness of untanned skin. Because sunless tanning is prevalent, it represents another important focus for intervention is amenable to appearance appeals.[78]

On the whole, these educational messages may, however, be based on an inaccurate assessment of the causes of skin cancer.[79] Although sunscreen use is important in reducing erythema (sunburn), clear evidence that it is associated with a reduction in melanoma or basal cell skin cancer is lacking, and the public may realize this. In the coming years, behavioral and psychosocial approaches will be important in addressing challenges on the horizon for skin cancer control. For example, the availability of genomic testing for melanoma may raise new questions on how to encourage sun protection in those who are tested to be genetically susceptible to melanoma or other skin cancers.[80]

Screening

Finally, the value of sun protection versus screening in melanoma control will have implications for the focus of behavioral intervention approaches, with both higher-risk and general population cohorts.[81] Secondary prevention is a potentially useful tool in the armamentarium against morbidity and mortality from skin cancer. Although there are no randomized trials supporting widespread population-based screening for melanoma, the idea of skin screening remains appealing for melanoma—a visible malignancy that appears to have mortality benefit when detected early. Persons with a family history of melanoma or with multiple or atypical moles, and those with a previous diagnosis of melanoma are candidates for intensive skin examination, either by themselves or by a physician.

Although physicians have been shown to diagnose melanoma at a thinner stage,[82] many more opportunities for physicians to provide skin cancer prevention counseling exist as only 1.5% of adults and fewer adolescents received such counseling. Although the evidence for the value of a melanoma screening program has been found to be insufficient by the US Preventive Services Task Force,[83] Geller and colleagues[84] are concerned that we may never have the randomized trial evidence that would convince individuals that screening will prevent mortality from melanoma. They point out the low screening rates in the population and suggest a rational program to find those at highest risk. In the first place, a baseline total skin examination of all white men 50 years and older seems rational. These are the individuals who most often have deep lesions and who die from melanoma; half of the melanoma-related deaths occur in this group. Geller and colleagues[84] lobby for expansion of public outreach, public and professional education and also legislative efforts.

Optimism is provided by Pennie and colleagues[85] who find that primary care providers are able to identify and treat melanomas appropriately—at almost the level of trained dermatologists. The barriers, however, are critical to consider: physicians need more changing rooms to facilitate full body examinations; there is no payment mechanism currently for a physician conducted skin examination; and there is little assistance for the uninsured.

SUMMARY

The many complexities described lead to difficulty when implementing skin cancer programs. Protection from UV radiation exposure—shade seeking, staying out of the sun during the peak hours of UV radiation, and wearing protective clothing—is likely to be effective. However, the use of any one of these preventive factors is infrequent. Current attempts to limit solar exposure through reduced exposure and sun protection are only partially successful. Despite extensive publicity campaigns, rates of melanoma in Australia are still increasing. In Queensland, the most recent analysis shows that invasive melanoma is increasing at a rate of 2.5 percent per year in males and 1.2 percent per year in females; with most of the increase among the thinner lesions, although rates appear to be stabilizing among those under 35 years old.[6] There is some evidence that individuals can be taught skin self-examination (SSE). The Check It Out Project has shown that individuals can be relatively easily trained to reliably examine their own skin.[86] Some evidence suggests that those who feel comfortable with SSE do better, and that might account for the difference in mortality (under study now).

Until we have better data on how to prevent skin cancer of all types, it makes sense to practice as much sun protection as possible (after getting that 15 minutes of UV exposure three times a week for vitamin D synthesis) and to practice SSE in combination with physician skin examination (either primary care practitioner or dermatologist) to evaluate any concerning skin lesions that may appear.

REFERENCES

1. Mouw T, Koster A, Wright ME, et al. Education and risk of cancer in a large cohort of men and women in the United States. PLoS ONE 2008;3:e3639.
2. Shack L, Jordan C, Thomson CS, et al. Variation in incidence of breast, lung and cervical cancer and malignant melanoma of the skin by socioeconomic group in England. BMC Cancer 2008;8:271.
3. Birch-Johansen F, Huilsom G, Kjaer T, et al. Social inequality and incidence of and survival from malignant melanoma in a population-based study in Denmark, 1994-2003. Eur J Cancer 2008;44:2043-9.
4. Parkin DM, Bray F, Ferlay J, et al. Global cancer statistics, 2002. CA Cancer J Clin 2005;55:74-108.
5. American Cancer Society. Cancer facts & figures 2008. Atlanta (GA): American Cancer Society; 2008.
6. Baade P, Coory M. Trends in melanoma mortality in Australia: 1950-2002 and their implications for melanoma control. Aust N Z J Public Health 2005;29(4): 383-6.
7. Qin J, Berwick M, Ashbolt R, et al. Quantifying the change of melanoma incidence by Breslow thickness. Biometrics 2002;58(3):665-70.
8. Welch HG, Woloshin S, Schwartz LM. Skin biopsy rates and incidence of melanoma: population based ecological study. BMJ 2005;331:481.
9. Gandini S, Sera F, Cattaruzza MS, et al. Meta-analysis of risk factors for cutaneous melanoma: II. Sun exposure. Eur J Cancer 2005;41(1):45-60.
10. Elwood JM, Jopson J. Melanoma and sun exposure: an overview of published studies. Int J Cancer 1997; 73:198-203.
11. Nelemans PJ, Rampen FH, Ruiter DJ, et al. An addition to the controversy on sunlight exposure and melanoma risk: a meta-analytical approach. J Clin Epidemiol 1995;48(11):1331-42.
12. Armstrong BK. Epidemiology of malignant melanoma: intermittent or total accumulated exposure to the sun? J Dermatol Surg Oncol 1988;14(8): 835-49.
13. Berwick M, Chen YT. Reliability of reported sunburn history in a case-control study of cutaneous malignant melanoma. Am J Epidemiol 1995;141(11): 1033-7.
14. Whiteman D, Green A. Melanoma and sunburn. Cancer Causes Control 1994;5(6):564-72.
15. MacKie RM, Aitchison T. Severe sunburn and subsequent risk of primary cutaneous malignant melanoma in Scotland. Br J Cancer 1982;46(6):955-60.
16. Grob JJ, Gouvernet J, Aymar D, et al. Count of benign melanocytic nevi as a major indicator of risk for nonfamilial nodular and superficial spreading melanoma. Cancer 1990;66(2):387-95.
17. Thomas NE, Edmiston SN, Alexander A. Number of nevi and early-life ambient UV exposure are associated with BRAF-mutant melanoma. Cancer Epidemiol Biomarkers Prev 2007;16(5):991-7.
18. Whiteman DC, Watt P, Purdie DM, et al. Melanocytic nevi, solar keratoses, and divergent pathways to cutaneous melanoma. J Natl Cancer Inst 2003; 95(11):806-12.
19. Berwick M. Are tanning beds "safe"? Human studies of melanoma. Pigment Cell Melanoma Res 2008; 21(5):517-9.
20. The International Agency for Research on Cancer Working Group on artificial ultraviolet (UV) light and skin cancer. Int J Cancer 2006;120:1116-22.
21. Veierød M, Weiderpass E, Thöm M, et al. A prospective study of pigmentation, sun exposure, and risk of cutaneous malignant melanoma in women. J Natl Cancer Inst 2003;95(20):1530-8.
22. Massi D, Carli P, Franchi A, et al. Naevus-associated melanomas: cause or chance? Melanoma Res 1999; 9(1):85-91.
23. Skender-Kalnenas TM, English DR, Heenan PJ. Benign melanocytic lesions: risk markers or precursors of cutaneous melanoma? J Am Acad Dermatol 1995;33(6):1000-7.
24. Olsen CM, Zens MS, Stukel TA, et al. Nevus density and melanoma risk in women: A pooled analysis to test the divergent pathway hypothesis. Int J Cancer 2008;124(4):937-44.
25. Chang YM, Newton-Bishop JA, Bishop DT, et al. A pooled analysis of melanocytic nevus phenotype and the risk of cutaneous melanoma at different latitudes. Int J Cancer 2008;124(2):420-8.
26. Gandini S, Sera F, Cattaruzza MS, et al. Meta-analysis of risk factors for cutaneous melanoma: I. Common and atypical naevi. Eur J Cancer 2005; 41(1):28-44.
27. Greene MH, Fraumeni JJ. The hereditary variant of malignant melanoma. In: Clark WH, Goldman LI, Mastrangelo MJ, editors. Human malignant melanoma. New York: Grune & Stratton; 1979, p. 139-66.
28. Kopf AW, Hellman LJ, Rogers GS, et al. Familial malignant melanoma. J Am Med Assoc 1986;256: 1915-9.
29. Ford D, Bliss JM, Swerdlow AJ, et al. Risk of cutaneous melanoma associated with a family history of the disease. Int J Cancer 1995;62:377-81.
30. Fitzpatrick TB. The validity and practicality of sun-reactive skin types I through VI. Arch Dermatol 1988;124:869-71.
31. Rampen FH, Fleuren BA, de Boo TM, et al. Unreliability of self-reported burning tendency and tanning ability. Arch Dermatol 1988;124(6):885-8.

32. Raimondi S, Sera F, Gandini S, et al. MC1R variants, melanoma and red hair color phenotype: a meta-analysis. Int J Cancer 2008;122(12):2753–60.

33. Gudbjartsson DF, Sulem P, Stacey SN, et al. MC1R. Nat Genet 2008;40(7):886–91.

34. Brown KM, Macgregor S, Montgomery GW, et al. Common sequence variants on 20q11.22 confer melanoma susceptibility. Nat Genet 2008;40(7):838–40.

35. Kertat K, Rosdahl I, Sun XF, et al. The Gln/Gln genotype of XPD codon 751 as a genetic marker for melanoma risk and Lys/Gln as an important predictor for melanoma progression: a case control study in the Swedish population. Oncol Rep 2008;20(1):179–83.

36. Millikan RC, Hummer A, Begg C, et al. Polymorphisms in nucleotide excision repair genes and risk of multiple primary melanoma: the Genes Environment and Melanoma Study. Carcinogenesis 2006;27(3):610–8.

37. Kadekaro AL, Wakamatsu K, Ito S, et al. Cutaneous photoprotection and melanoma susceptibility: reaching beyond melanin content to the frontiers of DNA repair. Front Biosci 2006;11:2157–73.

38. Han J, Colditz GA, Hunter DJ. Lack of associations of selected variants in genes involved in cell cycle and apoptosis with skin cancer risk. Cancer Epidemiol Biomarkers Prev 2006;15(3):592–3.

39. Berwick M, Orlow I, Hummer AJ, et al. The prevalence of CDKN2A germ-line mutations and relative risk for cutaneous malignant melanoma: an international population-based study. Cancer Epidemiol Biomarkers Prev 2006;15(8):1520–5.

40. Kefford R, Bishop JN, Tucker M, et al. Genetic testing for melanoma. Lancet Oncol 2002;3(11):653–4.

41. Armstrong BK, Kricker A, English DR. Sun exposure and skin cancer. Australas J Dermatol 1997;38(Suppl 1):S1–6.

42. American Cancer Society. Available at: www.cancer.org. Accessed 2009.

43. Hall HI, May DS, Lew RA, et al. Sun protection behaviors of the U.S. white population. Prev Med 1997;26(4):401–7.

44. Koh HK, Bak SM, Geller AC, et al. Sunbathing habits and sunscreen use among white adults: results of a national survey. Am J Public Health 1997;87(7):1214–7.

45. Coups EJ, Manne SL, Heckman CJ. Multiple skin cancer risk behaviors in the U.S. population. Am J Prev Med 2008;34(2):87–93.

46. Dobbinson SJ, Wakefield MA, Jamsen KM, et al. Weekend sun protection and sunburn in Australia trends (1987-2002) and association with SunSmart television advertising. Am J Prev Med 2008;34(2):94–101.

47. Montague M, Borland R, Sinclair C. Slip! Slop! Slap! and SunSmart, 1980-2000: Skin cancer control and 20 years of population-based campaigning. Health Educ Behav 2001;28(3):290–305.

48. Stanton WR, Moffatt J, Clavarino A. Community perceptions of adequate levels and reasons for skin protection. Behav Med 2005;31(1):5–15.

49. Saraiya M, Glanz K, Briss P. Preventing skin cancer: findings of the Task Force on Community Preventive Services on reducing exposure to ultraviolet light. MMWR Recomm Rep 2003;52:1–12.

50. Rutten L, Hesse BW, Moser RP, et al. Public understanding of cancer prevention, screening, and survival: Comparison with state-of-science evidence for colon, skin, and lung cancer. J Cancer Educ, in press.

51. Geller AC, Emmons KM, Brooks DR, et al. A randomized trial to improve early detection and prevention practices among siblings of melanoma patients. Cancer 2006;107(4):806–14.

52. Mayer JA, Lewis EC, Eckhardt L, et al. Promoting sun safety among zoo visitors. Prev Med 2001;33(3):162–9.

53. Weinstock MA, Rossi JS, Redding CA, et al. Randomized controlled community trial of the efficacy of a multicomponent stage-matched intervention to increase sun protection among beachgoers. Prev Med 2002;35(6):84–92.

54. Buller DB, Andersen PA, Walkosz BJ, et al. Randomized trial testing a worksite sun protection program in an outdoor recreation industry. Health Educ Behav 2005;32:514–35.

55. Glanz K, Geller AC, Shigaki D, et al. A randomized trial of skin cancer prevention in aquatics settings: the Pool Cool program. Health Psychol 2002;21(6):579–87.

56. Gorham ED, Mohr SB, Garland CF, et al. Do sunscreens increase risk of melanoma in populations residing at higher latitudes? Ann Epidemiol 2007;17(12):956–63.

57. Vainio H, Miller AB, Bianchini F. An international evaluation of the cancer-preventive potential of sunscreens. Int J Cancer 2000;88(5):838–42.

58. Autier P, Boniol M, Dore JF. Sunscreen use and increased duration of intentional sun exposure: still a burning issue. Int J Cancer 2007;121(1):2755–9.

59. Diffey BL. Sunscreens and melanoma: the future looks bright. Br J Dermatol 2005;153(2):378–81.

60. Gallagher RP, Rivers JK, Lee TK. Broad-spectrum sunscreen use and the development of new nevi in white children: a randomized controlled trial. JAMA 2000;283(22):2955–60.

61. Whiteman DC, Brown RM, Purdie DM, et al. Melanocytic nevi in very young children: the role of phenotype, sun exposure, and sun protection. J Am Acad Dermatol 2005;52(1):40–7.

62. van der Pols JC, Xu C, Boyle GM, et al. Expression of p53 tumor suppressor protein in sun-exposed skin and associations with sunscreen use and time spent outdoors: a community-based study. Am J Epidemiol 2006;163(11):982–8.

63. Bauer J, Büttner P, Wiecker TS, et al. Effect of sunscreen and clothing on the number of melanocytic nevi in 1,812 German children attending day care. Am J Epidemiol 2005;161(7):620–7.

64. English DR, Milne E, Simpson JA. Sun protection and the development of melanocytic nevi in children. Cancer Epidemiol Biomarkers Prev 2005; 14(12):2873–6.

65. English DR, Milne E, Simpson JA. Ultraviolet radiation at places of residence and the development of melanocytic nevi in children (Australia). Cancer Causes Control 2006;17(1):103–7.

66. Autier P, Doré JF, Cattaruzza MS, et al. Sunscreen use, wearing clothes, and number of nevi in 6- to 7-year-old European children. European Organization for Research and Treatment of Cancer Melanoma Cooperative Group. J Natl Cancer Inst 1998; 90(24):1873–80.

67. Gallagher RP, Elwood JM, Yang CP. Is chronic sunlight exposure important in accounting for increases in melanoma incidence? Int J Cancer 1989;44(5):813–5.

68. Diffey B. Do white British children and adolescents get enough sunlight? BMJ 2005;331:3–4.

69. Hiom S. Public awareness regarding UV risks and vitamin D—the challenges for UK skin cancer prevention campaigns. Prog Biophys Mol Biol 2006;92(1):161–6.

70. Working Group of the Australian and New Zealand Bone and Mineral Society, Endocrine Society of Australia and Osteoporosis Australia. Vitamin D and adult bone health in Australia and New Zealand: a position statement. Med J Aust 2005;182(6): 281–5.

71. Breitbart EW, Greinert R, Volkmer B. Effectiveness of information campaigns. Prog Biophys Mol Biol 2006; 92(1):167–72.

72. Brooks KR, Brooks DR, Hufford D, et al. Are television stations and weather pages still reporting the UV index? A national media follow-up study. Arch Dermatol 2005;141(4):526.

73. Dixon H, Armstrong B. The UV index. Report of a national workshop on its role in sun protection. Sydney: NSW Cancer Council and Anti-Cancer Council of Victoria; 1999.

74. Arthey S, Clarke VA. Suntanning and sun protection: a review of the psychological literature. Soc Sci Med 1995;40(2):265–74.

75. Berwick M, Fine JA, Bolognia JL. Sun exposure and sunscreen use following a community skin cancer screening. Prev Med 1992;21(3):302–10.

76. Grob JJ, Guglielmina C, Gouvernet J, et al. Study of sunbathing habits in children and adolescents: application to the prevention of melanoma. Dermatology 1993;186(2):94–8.

77. Jackson KM, Aiken LS. A psychosocial model of sun protection and sunbathing in young women: the impact of health beliefs, attitudes, norms, and self-efficacy for sun protection. Health Psychol 2000; 19(5):469–78.

78. Hoerster KD, Mayer JA, Woodruff SI, et al. The influence of parents and peers on adolescent indoor tanning behavior: findings from a multi-city sample. J Am Acad Dermatol 2007;57(6):990–7.

79. Young AR, Potten CS, Chadwick CA, et al. Photoprotection and 5-MOP photochemoprotection from UVR-induced DNA damage in humans: the role of skin type. J Invest Dermatol 1991;97(5):942–8.

80. Hay JL, Meischke HW, Bowen DJ, et al. Anticipating dissemination of cancer genomics in public health: a theoretical approach to psychosocial and behavioral challenges. Ann Behav Med 2007;34(3): 275–86.

81. Wartman D, Weinstock M. Are we overemphasizing sun avoidance in protection from melanoma? Cancer Epidemiol Biomarkers Prev 2008;17(3):469–70.

82. Epstein DS, Lange JR, Gruber SB, et al. Is physician detection associated with thinner melanomas? JAMA 1999;281(7):640–3.

83. US Preventive Services Task Force. Recommendations and rationale for screening for skin cancer. Am J Prev Med 2001;203(Suppl):44–6.

84. Geller AC, Sober AJ, Zhang Z, et al. Strategies for improving melanoma education and screening for men age > or = 50 years: findings from the American Academy of Dermatological National Skin Cancer Screening Program. Cancer 2002;95(7):1554–61.

85. Pennie ML, Soon SL, Risser JB, et al. Melanoma outcomes for Medicare patients: association of stage and survival with detection by a dermatologist vs a non-dermatologist. Arch Dermatol 2007;143(4):488–94.

86. Weinstock MA, Risica PM, Martin RA, et al. Melanoma early detection with thorough skin self-examination: the "Check It Out" randomized trial. Am J Prev Med 2007;32(6):517–24.

Index

Note: Page numbers of article titles are in **boldface** type.

A

Acne vulgaris
  and adherence behavior, 115–116
Acute lymphoblastic leukemia
  and atopic dermatitis, 142
Addiction
  to ultraviolet tanning, 109–111
Addiction and dependence
  models of, 110–111
Adherence behavior
  and corticosteroids, 115–117
  and dermatologic medication, 113–118
  and doctor-patient relationship, 116–117
  and lifestyle factors, 117
  and patient and caregiver education, 117–118
  and patient preferences, 117
  and psychosocial factors, 118
  and social cognitive theory, 114–115
  and studies in dermatology, 115–117
  studies to improve, 117–118
  and topical dermatologic medication, 113–118
  and treatment for acne vulgaris, 115–116
  and treatment for atopic dermatitis, 116–117
  and treatment for psoriasis, 115
  and written action plans, 117–118
AIDS advocacy
  and consumer-driven research, 177
Allergic rhinitis
  and atopic dermatitis, 141
Asthma
  and atopic dermatitis, 141
Atopic dermatitis
  and acute lymphoblastic leukemia, 142
  and adherence behavior, 116–117
  and allergic rhinitis, 141
  and asthma, 141
  and comorbidities, 141–142
  and herpes, 142
  and infections, 141–142
  and malignancies, 142

B

Basal cell carcinoma
  and comorbidities, 143
  and tanning, 150
BCC. See *Basal cell carcinoma.*
The benefits and risks of ultraviolet tanning and its
  alternatives:

The role of prudent sun exposure, **149–154**
Breast cancer advocacy
  and consumer-driven research, 177–178
Burdon of illness
  and skin disease, 99

C

CAGE criteria
  and ultraviolet tanning addiction, 110–111
CAM. See *Complementary and alternative medicine.*
Cardiovascular disease
  and psoriasis, 138–139
Cell cycle genes
  and melanoma, 207
Childhood vaccine refusal
  and consumer influence, 178
Clinical resources
  on the Internet, 194–195
Community-based surveys, 129
Comorbidities in dermatology, **137–147**
  and atopic dermatitis, 141–142
  and depression, 143–144
  and nonmelanoma skin cancer, 142–143
  and psoriasis, 137–141
  and vitiligo, 142
Complementary and alternative medicine
  and consumer influence, 178
Consumer-driven research
  and AIDS, 177
  and breast cancer, 177–178
  and prostate cancer, 178
Consumer empowerment in dermatology, **177–183**
Consumer influence
  and childhood vaccine refusal, 178
  on complementary and alternative medicine, 178
  on direct advertising, 178
  on study designs, 178–179
Contact dermatitis
  and nickel allergy, 155–160
Corticosteroids
  and adherence behavior, 115–117

D

Dehydroxyacetone
  and sunless tanning, 151
Depression
  as a comorbidity in dermatology, 143–144
Dermatologic medication adherence, **113–120**

Dermatol Clin 27 (2009) 215–218
doi:10.1016/S0733-8635(09)00009-6
0733-8635/09/$ – see front matter © 2009 Elsevier Inc. All rights reserved.

derm.theclinics.com

Dermatology Internet resources, **193–199**
Dermatology registries
    cancer registries, 187
    registries of procedures, 188–189
    registries of rare disorders, 187–188
    treatment registries, 189
DHA. See *Dehydroxyacetone.*
Direct advertising
    and consumer influence, 178
DNA repair genes
    and melanoma, 207
Doctor-patient relationship
    and adherence behavior, 116–117

E

Ear piercing
    and nickel allergy, 156
Educational materials
    on the Internet, 194, 196, 198
Evidence-based medicine resources
    on the Internet, 197–198

F

Facebook
    and evidence-based medicine resources, 198
    and health information, 133, 135

G

Google
    and health care information, 179–180

H

Health belief model
    of adherence behavior, 114–115
Health care inequities
    and melanoma, 104
    and minorities, 103–106
    and skin cancer, 104
    solutions for, 104–106
    in the United States, 103–104
Health care inequities: An introduction for
    dermatology providers, **103–107**
Health information
    on the Internet, 133–135
Health-related quality of life
    and comorbidities in dermatology, 143–144
Herpes
    and atopic dermatitis, 142
    and public health, 99
HRQOL. See *Health-related quality of life.*
Human immunodeficiency virus
    and psoriasis, 140–141

Human papilloma virus
    and public health, 99

I

Indoor tanning, 109–111, 149–152
Infections
    and atopic dermatitis, 141–142
    and psoriasis, 140–141
The Internet
    clinical resources on, 194–195
    and consumer influence, 179–180
    and dermatology consumers, 180–181
    dermatology resources on, 193–198
    educational materials on, 194, 196, 198
    evidence-based medicine resources on, 197–198
    and health information, 133–135
    and open access dermatology journals, 194

K

Kaposi's sarcoma
    and darker skin, 104

L

Lifestyle factors
    and adherence behavior, 117

M

Mail-based surveys, 123
Malignancies
    and atopic dermatitis, 142
    and psoralen plus ultraviolet A, 139–140
    and psoriasis, 139–140
Manuscript review, 201–203
    detecting plagiarism and duplicate publications,
        203
    principles of, 201–202
Manuscripts
    abstract, 202
    components of, 202–203
    discussion section, 203
    initial review of, 202
    introduction, 202
    methods section, 202–203
    online appendix, 203
    reference section, 203
    results section, 203
    title page, 202
Medical consumers, 177–181
Medical registry
    and dermatology research, 185–189
    essential requirements for, 186
    and peculiarities of dermatology, 186–187
Melanocytic nevi
    and melanoma, 206

Melanoma
    and cell cycle genes, 207
    and childhood education, 208
    and classification of skin types, 207
    and clothing as protection, 209
    and darker skin, 104
    and DNA repair genes, 207
    and education for high-risk populations, 208–209
    and educational strategies, 208–209
    epidemiology of, 205–207
    and family history, 206–208
    and gene-environment interaction, 207
    and health care inequities, 104
    and interventions in high-risk environments, 209
    and melanocytic nevi, 206
    and phenotypic characteristics, 207
    and physician counseling, 208
    and pigmentation genes, 207
    and public health, 207–210
    risk factors for, 205–206
    screening for, 211
    and sun exposure, 206
    and sun exposure behavior, 211
    and sunscreen, 209
    and the ultraviolet index, 210
    and ultraviolet radiation, 206
    and variation in susceptibility genes, 207
    and vitamin D and sun exposure, 209–210
Melanoma epidemiology and public health, **205–214**
Microblogging
    and health information, 135
Minorities
    and health care inequities, 103–106
MySpace
    and health information, 133, 135

N

Nickel
    in consumer items, 159–160
Nickel allergy
    barriers against, 158–159
    clinical presentation of, 156–157
    diagnosis and treatment of, 158
    immunology and genetics of, 155–156
    from implanted metal devices, 157–158
    prevalence of, 155
    prevention of, 158–159
    risk factors for, 156
NMSC. See *Nonmelanoma skin cancer*.
Nonmelanoma skin cancer
    and comorbidities, 142–143

O

Open access dermatology journals
    on the Internet, 194

P

Patient and caregiver education
    and adherence behavior, 117–118
Patient-based surveys, 128–129
Patient preferences
    and adherence behavior, 117
Physician-based surveys, 129
Pigmentation genes
    and melanoma, 207
Poverty
    and health care inequities, 104
Prevention of nickel allergy: The case for regulation?
    155–161
Primary health care
    and skin disease, 100
Prostate cancer advocacy
    and consumer-driven research, 178
Psoralen plus ultraviolet A
    and malignancies, 139–140
Psoriasis
    and adherence behavior, 115
    and cardiovascular disease, 138–139
    and comorbidities, 137–141
    and human immunodeficiency virus, 140–141
    and infections, 140–141
    and malignancies, 139–140
Psoriatic arthritis, 137–138
Psychosocial factors
    and adherence behavior, 118
Public health
    and melanoma education, 207–210
    and skin disease, 99–100

Q

Quality of life
    and comorbidities in dermatology, 143–144
Questionnaires, 121–129

R

Registry research in dermatology, **185–191**
Reviewing dermatology manuscripts and
    publications, **201–204**

S

SCC. See *Squamous cell carcinoma*.
Second Life
    and health information, 135
Skin aging
    and ultraviolet light, 150
Skin cancer
    and health care disparities, 104
    and stage at detection, 104
    and ultraviolet tanning addiction, 109–110

Skin disease
    and burden of illness, 99
    and primary health care, 100
    public health perspective of, 99–100
    and public healthy neglect, 99–100
Skin disease: A neglected public health problem,
    99–101
Social cognitive theory
    and adherence behavior, 114–115
Social Internet sites as a source of public health
    information, **133–136**
Social media marketing
    and health information, 133
Social networking Web sites
    and health information, 133–134
Squamous cell carcinoma
    and comorbidities, 143
    and tanning, 150
SRD. See *Substance-related disorder.*
Study designs
    consumer influence on, 178–179
Substance-related disorder
    and ultraviolet light, 111
Sunless tanning, 151
Sunscreen
    and melanoma, 209
Survey design
    and limiting error, 128
    and survey format, 124–125
    and survey questions, 125–128
Survey questions, 125–128
Survey research
    basics of, 121–122
    and community-based surveys, 129
    and designing surveys, 124–128
    and face-to-face interviews, 123
    guidelines for, 121–124
    and mail-based surveys, 123
    and patient-based surveys, 128–129
    and physician-based surveys, 129
    and publication, 128
    and residency- and fellowship-based surveys, 129
    and response rates, 122–123
    and sampling methods, 122
    and telephone surveys, 123
    and types of surveys, 123–124
    and Web-based surveys, 124
Survey research in dermatology: Guidelines for
    success, **121–131**
Susceptibility genes
    and melanoma, 207

T

T-cell lymphoma
    and darker skin, 104
Tanning, 109–111, 149–152

    addiction to, 110–111
    and basal cell carcinoma, 150
    health benefits of, 149–150
    health risks of, 150–151
    and squamous cell carcinoma, 150
    and vitamin D production, 150
Teledermatologists versus clinic-based
    dermatologists
    diagnostic agreement rates between, 164–169
    intragroup diagnostic agreement between, 165,
        169
Teledermatology
    diagnostic accuracy of, 165–172
    and management plan agreement rates, 172
Teledermatology: A review of reliability and accuracy
    of diagnosis and management, **163–176**
Telemedicine, 163–173
Telephone surveys, 123
Topical dermatologic medication
    and adherence behavior, 113–118
Twitter
    and health information, 135

U

Ultraviolet index
    and melanoma, 210
Ultraviolet light
    behavioral responses to, 111
    and skin aging, 150
    and skin cancer, 150
    and substance-related disorder, 111
Ultraviolet tanning addiction, **109–112**
    and CAGE criteria, 110–111
    and skin cancer, 109–110
    survey studies on, 111
UVI. See *Ultraviolet index.*

V

Vitamin D production
    and sun exposure, 209–210
    and tanning, 150
Vitiligo
    and comorbidities, 142

W

WAPs. See *Written action plans.*
Web-based surveys, 124
Written action plans
    and adherence behavior, 117–118

Y

You-Tube
    and health information, 134–135

Moving?

Make sure your subscription moves with you!

To notify us of your new address, find your **Clinics Account Number** (located on your mailing label above your name), and contact customer service at:

E-mail: elspcs@elsevier.com

800-654-2452 (subscribers in the U.S. & Canada)
314-453-7041 (subscribers outside of the U.S. & Canada)

Fax number: 314-523-5170

Elsevier Periodicals Customer Service
11830 Westline Industrial Drive
St. Louis, MO 63146

*To ensure uninterrupted delivery of your subscription, please notify us at least 4 weeks in advance of move.

Printed and bound by CPI Group (UK) Ltd, Croydon, CR0 4YY

03/10/2024

01040361-0011